How To Survive Your Health Care

Carrie Bowers

Disclaimer: The author and the publisher have strived to ensure the
accuracy of the information contained within this book, however, the
health care field is ever changing. This book is intended as a guide to
navigating the health care system and not as a substitute for a positive
relationship with a licensed health care provider.

Dedication

This book is dedicated in loving memory of my parents, Curtis and Dorothy Bowers.

Their unconditional love, support and guidance provided me with the courage and strength to pursue my dreams. They taught me to be persistent and to stand firm in my convictions. Through their example, I learned to advocate for myself and others. I thank them for a lifetime of wonderful lessons, experiences and memories.

Acknowledgements:

I would like to thank the many friends, colleagues, patients and families who provided me with their support, encouragement and stories during the writing of this book.

Artwork and design TM- Creative Life Solutions, LLC

Logo design TM-Creative Life Solutions, LLC

Artwork and cover design by Pam McClung

Interior design and typesetting by Pam McClung

Logo design and content consultant - Lisa Applegate-Lewis, MSW-LISW

Editing and Content Review by: Gwen Valore and Ruth Chavez, MS, RN, CNP

Creative Life Solutions Consulting, LLC is a subsidiary of Bowers and Associates, LLC

Table of Contents

Introduction

Welcome to Creative Life Solutions' *How to Survive Your Health Care*. I would like to take this opportunity to introduce our company, explain why we started this venture and how this book may help you navigate not only the health care system, but also life's inevitabilities.

As an experienced nurse working in the traditional setting of a hospital emergency room, I see patients coming into the health care system virtually unprepared to deal with decisions they are being asked to make. There are also patients coming into the system with multiple health and social issues that the health care system is often unable to address adequately. Patients need honest information in a way that they can understand and apply to their own personal situations. Because of the constraints imposed by the corporate environment of health care, many patients pass through the system having no control over the outcome of their health, wellness, life and death.

Another motivation for starting Creative Life Solutions™ arose from a personal experience. As I guided my mother through the last stages of her life, I realized the importance of having a Health Advocate, a person who not only knows the system, but the terminology necessary to navigate the health care field and guide not only how we live, but also how we approach our final days of life.

While most health care professionals have good intentions and strive to provide recommended health care, they have had to change their practice to accommodate the challenges of dealing with insurance companies, lawyers and economic downturns. Because of these constraints, health care practitioners may not have the time, resources or courage to deal with all the problems that patients and their families experience. Creative Life Solutions™ represents you and/or your family members. We are not restricted by corporate restraints, and we facilitate systems and processes for you to insure that your health care and life planning needs are met.

Because Creative Life Solutions™ is a private pay company, we work for you. We do not represent insurance companies, hospitals, nursing homes or physicians. We help you and your family to work with the above groups to facilitate safe and adequate health care and life care. With the recent and future changes in the economy and health care, it is going to become increasingly difficult for the health care system to meet all the needs of their patient populations. Creative Life Solutions™ will provide a bridge for you and your loved ones that will aid in your navigation of the health care system.

This book is one section of that bridge. While we realize that not everyone can afford a Health Advocate, a health coach and/or a life care manager, we feel passionately that everyone should have some knowledge, power and control over the health and life care decisions that he faces throughout the course of life. This book provides tips to advocate for yourself and family members. It also provides ideas and solutions for common diseases and health issues. And finally, some of the basic steps needed to insure the care management needs of you and your family will be discussed.

Chapter 1

What is a Health Advocate, and Why Do I Need One?

Health advocacy is a term that can mean many things in today's health care environment. On a large scale, health advocacy is global, promoted by political action committees and grass root organizations. These groups work on a community, national or international level to effect change in the delivery of health care and health care systems. These are people who fight for better care, better insurance policies and try to guide change and legislation related to the delivery of health care.

Creative Life Solutions™ brings health advocacy to the individual and personal level. A personal Health Advocate is a person who represents the patient and family in many healthcare settings such as physicians' offices, hospitals, assisted living facilities and nursing homes. A personal Health Advocate provides you with guidance on how to get the most from your health care experience.

From a medical perspective, a Health Advocate acts as a translator, a mediator, a resource and most importantly, an additional safety net in the promotion of optimal health care. While health care providers generally are very diligent and strive to practice safely, health care is a system of checks and balances. When everyone does her job and performs her part, the results can be amazingly positive. However, when the checks and balances are not done correctly the results can be disastrous. We have all heard horror stories about people who have gone into the hospital and had the wrong body part operated on. This was simply a breakdown in the system. A Health Advocate can enhance this safety net by guiding the patient/family through the process through a thorough assessment, and provide education and information.

So let's look at ways a Health Advocate can be used:

Protecting your safety
As stated above, a Health Advocate is an additional thread that makes the medical safety net stronger. As a patient with perhaps little or no knowledge of how medical systems operate on a day-to-day basis, you may not know what questions to ask or what to look for in terms of the checks and balances of the health care system.

An example would be a patient who has never had surgery before. This patient goes into the surgery setting with his medical records, feeling confident that the surgeon he has spoken with is on the same page with what surgery is going to be performed. What the patient may not know is that the surgeon is probably doing several cases that day and they all look alike wearing cute little hairnets and oxygen masks. So part of the system includes making sure that the patient is wearing a wrist band that has his correct name and identifiers on it, and that everyone who has contact with that patient verifies the information. The patient should also be asked to mark the spot that is to be operated on, and this should be verified by the surgeon. Although there are many other checks that the surgeon and operating staff do behind the scenes to insure a patient's safety, if the patient goes in unaware of how the system works and just trusts that the system will function properly, accidents may unfortunately happen. Therefore, whether it is surgery or a routine doctor's appointment, a Health Advocate can provide information to make sure that he knows what to expect.

Translating Complicated Information

While doctors and nurses try to speak in terms that patients can understand, the fact is that they often talk their own lingo. Many times patients and medical personnel just simply speak a different language. When patients and doctors don't take the time to understand each other, the result is increased medical costs related to unnecessary testing and treatment, misdiagnosis and elevated risks to patients. A personal Health Advocate takes the time to make sure that everyone is on the same page promoting a safer outcome.

Let's look at a typical breakdown in the communication process between a patient and doctor. A patient came into the emergency room complaining that she had a "spell" and did not know what caused it. The doctor assumed that the patient's "spell" meant that she got dizzy, felt sick and possibly had a loss of consciousness, because the last patient who told the doctor about a "spell" had those very symptoms. The doctor ordered blood work, an IV, a CAT scan, and an EKG. When the patient questioned the nurse why she was getting all of these tests, the nurse explained why the doctor had ordered the tests. The patient then stated, "All of this because my right knee gave out on me?" A Health Advocate works with both the patient and the doctor to make sure the communication process works as it should. We will discuss more examples in the following chapters.

Explaining the Diagnosis

When a patient goes to the doctor and is told she has diabetes, hypertension, cancer, etc. what does she really hear? It is amazing sometimes how our brains function under stress. Most patients faced with a new and/or potentially life threatening diagnosis will generally hear and understand part of what the medical professional has just told them. Some patients, because of the stress response, will hear nothing, will deny the diagnosis or will suffer some confusion as to what the diagnosis is or what it means to their overall health status. This problem tends to increase with age. A Health Advocate reinforces the information and helps guide the patient through the decision process, as well as, works with the medical professional to insure adequate understanding and treatment options.

I have experienced this phenomenon on many occasions throughout my personal life and nursing career. My father was diagnosed with colon cancer. He went through several tests and a rather long operation and radiation therapy. He never could admit to the fact that he had cancer. The doctor told him, my mother told him, and I told him, but he firmly denied having cancer, stating that the doctor had just found a little spot that needed to be taken off. If he had not had my mother and me with him, he may not have proceeded with the proper course of treatment. In the emergency room setting, I often hear doctors give the patient diagnosis and treatment options, yet when I go into the room to do the discharge or admission, the patient will ask why the doctor has not told him what is wrong. This happens because when faced with a stressful situation, people tend to go into a protective mode and some information which is perceived as threatening or damaging gets blocked out.

A personal Health Advocate gently guides the patient through the blockage and personalizes the information to insure a better understanding and outcome.

Coordinating Care Givers
Often when we enter into the health care system, we are exposed to a number of different care providers.You may start with your family physician and then be referred to a specialist, surgeon, hospital internist and perhaps a rehabilitation facility. The ideal situation is that all these people communicate with each other. This rarely happens in the real world. The result can be exhausting, expensive and unsafe to you, the patient. Many times medical professionals feel that they need to order tests and medications to earn their keep and keep their patients happy. The result is that everyone you come in contact with orders something different, and if there is a breakdown in the communication channels, you end up with a lot of medications. Sometimes those medications are duplicated, unnecessary and, in the worst case scenario, unsafe.

A Health Advocate helps track and facilitate the communication between care providers. The Health Advocate also reviews your personal medical history and alerts you to potential problems and conflicts.

Disease Management

While medical professionals are usually pretty good at assessing, testing and prescribing according to your health needs, they often are not able to provide the education and regular attention to help you manage your disease processes on a day-to-day basis. There are several things that you need to take into consideration when managing your health or disease processes. You need to look at your total needs which include the medication component, lifestyle component and the daily management of your health and/or disease.

A Health Advocate helps you manage your disease on an ongoing basis. Your advocate acts as a health coach, resource person, educator, researcher and motivator for enacting a consistent and lifelong basis for health and lifestyle change.

Life Planning

Whether you're 18 or 118 it behooves you to plan for the unexpected. While we would all like to think that we are going to live forever and stay healthy, that often is not reality. If you were in an accident tomorrow who would know your wishes in regard to medical issues. We have heard the stories about families fighting over whether a loved one wanted certain medical procedures performed, life saving procedures or life sustaining measures taken. Just talking to your loved ones is not enough to insure that your wishes are carried out. You must have it in writing in legal form recognized by the medical community and updated regularly.

A Health Advocate guides you through the process, helps you make the decisions that are right for you and helps to insure that you keep your wishes up to date. Decisions change throughout the life span and should be updated accordingly. A discussion of the forms that are important to keep updated and the information that should be included on those forms will be addressed later.

Researching

Most people do not have the time to do the research required to make informed decisions in today's ever changing health care field. A personal Health Advocate does the research for you to save you valuable time and enhance your knowledge base of the available health care resources.

If you or a family member is facing a chronic or acute health issue, the last thing that you have time to do is spend endless hours at the library or online researching the latest treatments, medications, physicians and facilities. Many sources of information, especially on the web, are either financed by a company or organization that has a vested interest in convincing you that its services are valid. A Health Advocate helps you sift through the information, guides you to the most recent and reliable data, and works with you and your family to reach the decisions that will best serve your health care needs.

Benefit Analyzing

Many patients and families are unaware of the benefits and/or community services available to them. A Health Advocate can do a benefit analysis to see what benefits you qualify for. There are assessment tools used to determine what services, equipment and/or additional monies you or a family member may be entitled to receive. An advocate can also assist you in working with your insurance company to insure that you receive the maximum benefits from your policies.

Family Mediating

When faced with a health crisis, some families find that the communication process breaks down under the stress. The best way, of course, to avoid this scenario is to have advanced discussions with family and friends before a crisis situation arises. As stated in the life planning section, it is a good idea to have your wishes in writing and to talk with those around you regarding those wishes. In addition, make sure that those you share this information with either have or know where to find the copies of the documents.

In families where these difficult conversations are put off or family members are reluctant to proceed, a Health Advocate may step in to initiate the conversation. A client that came to us had this very problem. The client was a woman in her mid-sixties who was still very active and in good health. She wanted to talk to her adult children about what she wanted if her health should fail. The adult children kept telling her she was going to be around for a long time, and they could have this conversation later. This matter weighed heavily on the client's mind, and everyday she feared that something would happen, she would not be able to speak for herself, and no one would know or understand her wishes. Having felt that she had tried everything she could to communicate the importance of this conversation to her children, she called on us. In the advocate role, we were able to approach her children and bring all parties together for a successful resolution.

Another problem facing families may occur once a health care crisis hits. Whether advance directives are in place or not, conflict among family members over decision making may develop. Perhaps the family has not discussed the advance directives with the patient and is at odds with the patient's wishes. Other issues could involve sibling rivalries and blended families where there is a battle for control. A Health Advocate can work with all family members to aid in consensus and to keep the focus on what is in the best interest of the patient. Mediation provided by a Health Advocate can help in preventing family disharmony and promoting an outcome that everyone can agree on.

Facility Mediating
When a loved one enters a hospital or extended care facility, problems very often will occur. A Health Advocate can also help to mediate in these circumstances. Most problems revolve around the patient and/or family expectations and the actual delivery of care. A Health Advocate can help resolve the issues for you through educating you on the health care system and intervening on your behalf when you experience a problem.

For example, a client called late one night because her husband's condition changed a day after being admitted to an extended care facility. The wife had told the nurse that her husband was struggling with his breathing. The nurse stated that because he had pneumonia he would have trouble breathing and that there was nothing to be concerned about. The wife went home but continued to feel uncomfortable with her husband's condition. After receiving her call, we placed a call to the extended care facility and talked with the nurse taking care of the husband. As it turned out, the nurse was unfamiliar with the husband's entire medical history and the fact that he had a past history of cardiovascular disease. Our Advocate was able to enlighten the nurse about his history and expressed concern that the patient may be in congestive heart failure. Upon our Advocate's insistence, the nurse went back in to reassess the patient and ended up sending the patient back to the hospital for treatment of the congestive heart failure. Without intervention, there is very little doubt that this patient would have experienced a horrible, drowning type death that night. With the intervention, the patient was able to be kept comfortable and spend valuable time with his family. The patient did pass away a couple of days later, but comfortably and on his terms. According to the family, it allowed time for closure, greater comfort and a much more peaceful passing. To the patient and family it was a quality of life issue.

Whether it is medical management, nursing care or administrative policies that you may encounter issues with, a Health Advocate can help resolve those problems and provide guidance in order to achieve the maximum care and benefits from your care receiving experiences.

Assisting with transition
Whether for yourself or a loved one, a Health Advocate can be very helpful in easing the transitions that often accompany aging. If you, a parent and/or loved one is having trouble maintaining a home or is just simply ready for a down-size, a Health Advocate can guide you through the process. Through home safety assessments, transitional living location research and education on options, a Health Advocate can be an invaluable tool. If staying in the home setting is important,

a Health Advocate can assist in locating services and recommending home modifications to make the wish a reality.

Obtaining durable medical equipment

A Health Advocate can help you obtain durable medical equipment and services while optimizing your insurance benefits and minimizing your out of pocket costs. With the multitude of choices in durable medical equipment, it is helpful to have someone do the time consuming research and guide you through the process. Because Health Advocates help a wide array of clients, they have often already done the research and can provide you with a wealth of information very quickly.

Life coaching

A Health Advocate can also help navigate the stresses of life. As we all know, when stress enters our life, our health usually suffers. As our health suffers, our stressors start to multiply even faster. An Advocate can do a comprehensive assessment of stressors in your life and work with you to develop techniques and find alternative ways to reduce stress.

End of life counseling

End of life issues are areas that many people feel uncomfortable thinking and/or talking about, but they are inevitable. Ignoring them does not make them go away nor does it make easier for a loved one who may be facing the end of life. A Health Advocate can help individuals and families feel an increased sense of ease with these issues through education and counseling.

Decreasing medical costs and reducing hospital visits

Perhaps the most important function a Health Advocate can do for you is reduce your medical costs and hospital visits. Through advocating, educating and coordinating care, an Advocate can guide you into substantial health care savings.

Chapter 2

Who are Health Advocates, What Do They Do and How Do I Decide Which One to Hire?

Health Advocates can be nurses, social workers, physicians, nurse practitioners or physician assistants. Each profession can bring its own brand of advocacy to patients and families. They can practice in their own locality or they can work with patients and families across the country. Which one is right for you depends on what you need, want or prefer.

Physicians, nurse practitioners and physician assistants can prescribe and diagnose depending on the scope of their practice and the area in which they are advocating. Nurses and social workers assess, educate, manage and coordinate care, but do not diagnose or prescribe. Most advocates do not provide medical advice over the phone, but will help guide you along the decision making process through assessment and education.

What qualifications should you look for in a Health/Patient Advocate? You should take several things into consideration when selecting your advocate. First, decide what it is you want to achieve when working with someone who will be advocating for you. Physicians and physician assistants typically work only in the medical realm. Nurses, depending on their backgrounds, work in the medical area as well as care coordination. Social workers are generally very experienced in care coordination and community service referrals. All the professions listed above require licensing and you should make sure that your advocate has a license that is valid and current. Most states provide current licensure information on their licensing web pages. Health Advocates also may possess various certifications. Some certifications show if the advocate has done additional course work and/or testing. Perhaps the most important criteria when choosing an Advocate is how that person or company relates to you.

When you call a company or Advocate, pay close attention to how well you and the Advocate communicate from the start. Does the Advocate give you an opportunity to explain your needs, and are they able to repeat those needs back to you so that you feel comfortable they have understood what you are trying to achieve? Pay attention to your comfort level when making that first phone call. You and the Advocate will be working together very closely, and you will be sharing a great deal of personal information with this person. If you don't feel a sense of trust and ability to share with your Advocate, the advocacy process will be hampered and the results compromised.

When deciding on an Advocate, you will want to consider whether you want to work with a large or small company. You will also want to ask if you will be dealing with one person or multiple people. Also take into consideration what hours the company operates. If the company operates on an 8 to 5 schedule, you need to determine if that will fit your needs. From my experience in the medical field, most problems don't arise during normal business hours. Whether the company is large or small, we recommend that you work with the same advocate as much as possible. Generally, the more people that get involved the higher the risk of misunderstandings and process breakdowns.

The last two things to consider when selecting an Advocate is cost and length of time you want to employ someone. Most Advocates can do both short and long term assignments. Make sure that the company that you employ offers a plan that suits your needs.

Chapter 3

How to Advocate for Yourself

Creative Life Solutions™ understands that not everyone can or
wants to afford a Health Advocate, but it is our belief that everyone
should know the basics of health advocacy. Your health care dollars
are getting smaller and smaller. Health care reform, rising insurance
costs, decreased benefits and rising health care costs are a threat to
all of us. In order to insure that you get the most out of your health
care, some suggestions and guidance will be presented on how you
can achieve the safest and most cost effective way to accomplish your
health care goals.

Be an informed health care consumer
Let's face it, health care is an industry. Health care providers, pharmaceutical companies, hospitals, extended care facilities and insurance companies are all in business to make money. All have their
advantages and disadvantages. We as health care consumers need to
do our research to make sure that we are getting the service that best
fits our needs. It is not unusual to spend more time researching the
best cell phone prices and services than researching the best health
care choices. If we all looked at health care services in the same way
we shopped for a new car or the latest electronic gadgets, we would all
make better choices.

When researching your medical choices, make sure you know the
source of the information. If doing online research, determine who is
presenting the information. If researching a drug, is the site sponsored

by the pharmaceutical company or a competitor of the company? Either way can skew the information. Public libraries are often a good source of information and can often direct you to legitimate web sites. You can also talk to friends and family members to hear their experiences, but once again, look at the source and the motivation behind the advice.

Don't be afraid to ask questions

When you visit your health care provider, hospital, or extended care facility, don't be afraid to ask questions. Many patients say that their doctor doesn't have time to answer their questions. Patients need to look at medical professionals as they would any type of consumer product. After all, these people are in business, too. If your doctor does not allow you time to ask questions and/or take the time to explain things to you in a way that you can understand, perhaps you should consider finding another doctor. This rule also applies to hospital and/or extended care facility staff. Make sure that prior to any appointment you write down your list of questions, so that if you are stressed or feeling rushed, you won't forget what it is that you want to ask. Perhaps you have gone to your doctor, but it is not until you get home that you think of your questions, then what? First, you may want to call the office or facility to see if there is a nurse or assistant who can pull your information and assist you. If you still don't get the answers you are looking for, then request an appointment to have a more detailed conversation with the person in question. When making that appointment make sure that you let the scheduling staff know the purpose of your visit. Informing the scheduler that you have a list of questions will permit her to schedule the appropriate amount of time and allow the medical professional to have the records available to answer your questions.

So you have your questions in hand, you've got the appointment and the doctor has answered the questions, but you still don't quite understand. Many patients will say that they don't want to seem like a blithering idiot, so they walk out of the facility without the information they came in for. If the medical professional has used jargon that you didn't understand, or you don't feel that you understand what the

implications are, by all means, ask again. Most medical professionals
are good about explaining things from different perspectives, but if
you don't make it clear that you are not getting it, they will not know
to take a different approach. And finally, feel free to take notes and
request a printed copy of your medical records. When you have something in writing, you can then go home and read it over, look it up and
get a better understanding. It is your legal right to have a copy of your
records. Remember, it is your body and your health at stake!

Be prepared

Whether you are going to your family doctor, a specialist, hospital,
extended care facility or anything involving your health, have a
summary of your health history and a list of current medications with
you. You can make the list small and wallet sized so that you have it
with you at all times. It is also helpful to include in this list the time
of day you take the medications, dosages and how long you have been
taking them. Many medications have some rather significant side
effects, and it often helps the health care professional to have a time
line to see if your current problem may be related to your medications.
As a patient, it is also helpful if you are familiar with your medications and why you are taking each medication. It is surprising how
many patients that enter the health care system and have no idea the
names of their medications and/or why they are taking certain medications. Your list should include the following information:

MEDICAL HISTORY - List any diseases such as diabetes, high
blood pressure, cancer, pneumonia, chronic pain issues, mental health
issues, etc. and when they were diagnosed.

SURGICAL HISTORY - List surgeries, dates and hospitals where
surgeries were performed.

DRUG ALLERGIES - List all drug allergies, food allergies, material
allergies (ex: latex) and environmental allergies.

MEDICATIONS - List all prescription medications, over-the-counter medicines taken on a regular basis, herbal and dietary supplements. Make sure to list dosages, how often you take them, what time of day you take them and when you started taking them.

DOCTORS - List all health care providers that you see such as your family physician, specialist, and/or mental health professional.

INSURANCE - List your insurance companies and policy numbers.

Once you have your list completed make sure that you make several copies. Keep a copy or two in your purse or wallet, give one to your spouse or significant other, and make sure that your Durable Power of Attorney for Health Care has the list as well. Your list should be updated and new copies issued whenever there is a change in any of the information.

There is also a useful item called the Vial of Life. The Vial of Life is a little tube or envelop that contains the above mentioned information which can be placed in/on your refrigerator. Emergency personnel are trained to look in the refrigerator for this information when making an emergency call to a residence. Another good idea is to put an In Case of Emergency or I.C.E. number in your cell phone so if you are incapable of providing this information, emergency workers can retrieve it from your phone and notify your loved ones or Durable Power of Attorney for Health Care.

Don't be afraid to question
Questioning a medical professional is a little different from asking a question, but just as important. Using the cell phone analogy, when you walk into the cell phone store and the salesperson shows you a phone with fifty features that you don't need, you would question the salesperson to determine which are best for you. The same principle applies when dealing with medical professionals. You, as a consumer, have the right to know what your options are. You should be getting as much information about treatment options as possible. Let's look at some of the areas you might want to question:

MEDICATIONS:

What other options do I have besides taking a medication?

What are the potential side effects of the medication?

Are there lifestyle changes that I can make instead of taking a medication?

Are there cheaper medications that I can take that will provide the same benefits?

What are the long term effects of the medication?

Are there any natural remedies that would be just as effective?

SURGERIES:

What are the risks and benefits of the surgery?

Are there alternative treatments?

Can I get a second opinion and from whom?

How experienced is the surgeon in this procedure?

Your medical professional should feel comfortable answering these questions for you. If you feel that your care provider is not appreciative of your inquiries, perhaps it is time to find someone who is open to these discussions regarding your health care. Even in most medical emergencies there is time for you and/or your Durable Power of Attorney for Health Care to ask about all the options available.

Be an involved patient
So what happens once you get admitted to the hospital? Your vigilance should continue. Never assume that anyone cares about your health as much or more than you do. As stated before, most health care professionals are very conscientious and try to provide the best care possible, but there is a human factor that can come into play at any given time. Medical personnel have many of the same issues that their patients have, and this can, at times, affect their job performance. Nurses, physicians and social workers often have children, families, work long hours, get little sleep, have medical issues, financial issues, and a litany of other problems which may at times decrease their abilities and concentration. Once again, never be afraid to question. If you feel that you are getting the wrong medication, the wrong dosage, or the wrong procedure, speak up.

If you speak up and get ignored by the medical staff, but still feel that something is just not right, by all means take a time out and do not proceed with the treatment. You, as a patient, always have the right to refuse treatment, and should refuse if you feel that it is not right or you need more time to think about things. Explaining that you need time to think about things will let the medical professional know that you are involved and perhaps looking for more information.

If you feel that you are not getting the appropriate care, start with a polite and respectful conversation with the medical staff involved. If you are in the hospital and having trouble with pain control, call lights being answered, or any other care concerns, start with a conversation with your primary nurse. If this approach does not work, ask to speak with the charge nurse and continue working your way up the chain of command. In most facilities that chain of command starts with your primary nurse and then continues upward to the charge nurse, nursing supervisor, vice-president of nursing, hospital ombudsman. If you still feel that your concerns are not being addressed, ask to speak to the risk management department which will almost assuredly get someone's attention, but do this as a last resort when possible.

Take someone with you

If you find yourself in the hospital, chances are you are not feeling well, are being medicated and probably more than just a little stressed. This is when it is very helpful to have a friend or family member with you as much as possible. It is always a good idea to have someone who can pay attention when you can't. Make sure the people you have with you are knowledgeable about your condition and your wishes. Encourage those with you to take notes and keep track of medications, procedures and information that has been presented while you are unable or under the influence of medications or sedatives. That being said, allow yourself some time to rest, and allow some time for your friends or family members to rest. Depending on the facility or condition of the patient there may be restricted visiting hours established. These visiting hours are in place to allow the patients to get the rest required to heal. In this case, and if the facility is inflexible with the hours, have your family member leave a log in the room and encourage the staff to write entries into your log so you can have an accurate record of your care.

Be a financially responsible health care consumer

We would like to think that you can't put a price on good health care, but we all know that a lot of people know how to put a really big price on your health. As a health care consumer, you can often negotiate doctor fees, testing fees and hospital fees. Negotiating medical fees is not easy, but with persistence the cost savings can be substantial. Whether or not you have insurance, you can work to lower your health care costs.

It's amazing that people with insurance often get billed less than those without. The fact is that insurance companies negotiate fees with almost all health care outlets, and those outlets usually will accept reduced fees. For example, let's say that an insured patient has a surgery for which the hospital will bill $5,000. The insurance company says that the market average for that particular surgery is $3,000. The hospital will usually accept that amount for the surgery, and the patient will not be responsible for the other $2,000. Now, another patient comes through the door without insurance, and the hospital bills the same $5,000. Without the insurance company negotiating on this patient's behalf, this patient will indeed receive a bill for the full amount.

If you are an uninsured patient, you have the right to contact the billing office and request the same consideration. So how do you know what the market average is for health care procedures? Two reliable sources for information, once again, are the internet and the public library. Call the billing office and tell them that you have found that the average cost of the surgery is $3,000. Chances are they will tell you that they are unable to negotiate the price. This is where patience, persistence and doing your homework will pay off. Be patient and explain the sources of your information. If that tactic does not pay off, start working your way up the chain of command. Ask to speak to the person's supervisor and keep doing that until you get someone who will work with you.

Let's assume that you have been successful getting the price down, but you don't have $3,000 readily available. Now, you start to work on getting them to accept a payment plan. Many health care outlets will allow you to make monthly payments without interest. Often you can arrange payments as low as $10 per month. As long as a health care outlet sees that you are making an effort to pay, it will generally work with you.

The same applies if you do have insurance. As an insured patient, you may have a rather substantial deductible or co-pay. When you submit the bill to your insurance company, they will usually send you an Explanation of Benefits (referred to as an E.O.B.). The E.O.B will include the amount billed, the amount the insurance company would cover if your deductible were met and the amount applied to your deductible. Once again, there is a difference between the amount they will cover and the amount you are billed. Call the business office of the care facility and start your negotiations to lower the remainder of the bill.

What happens when you don't have insurance and have very few resources, can you still get health care? Well, it is not always easy, but it is possible. You do have several options available depending on your individual situation. The best approach to making sure that you have options where your health care is concerned, is to be proactive and explore your choices prior to needing health care services.

If you don't have a job, or have a low paying job without insurance, there are numerous public programs available. These programs are generally available through your state's department of jobs and family services. Most communities also have free clinics available, and it is useful to know where these clinics are prior to needing them. Hospitals also have social workers and case managers who can provide you with additional resources for financial assistance. If you need emergency or hospital services, go to the nearest emergency room. Emergency rooms are required to treat patients regardless of their insurance status. That being said, part of being a financially responsible health care consumer is to use emergency services responsibly. Every day, emergency rooms across the country are overwhelmed with non-emergencies such as pregnancy tests, colds, minor sore throats, etc. Inappropriate emergency service use is bogging down the system, delaying care to the more critical patients and costing every health care consumer.

If you have lost your job and insurance, one option is to apply for your company's COBRA plan. Often this is too pricey for most people who have just lost a job. Another option is to look for a private, individual plan. Once again, you can go online and compare private plans or find a reliable insurance agent that can do the shopping for you. The advantages of the individual plans are that they are generally cheaper than COBRA premiums, are usually tax deductible, and they prevent a catastrophic hit to your bank account and credit score. The disadvantages are that they are more difficult to afford if you have pre-existing conditions, and they usually come with much higher deductibles. When you compare a $5,000 deductible with a $50,000 dollar hospital bill, the answer becomes a little clearer.

Let your actions be seen and your voice be heard

Thus far, we have discussed ways to advocate for yourself within the health care system. Advocating for yourself also includes being aware of the struggles and changes taking place, and the impact that you can have on the future of health care. Regardless of your opinions on health care reform, it is vitally important that we make ourselves aware of the trends, the proposals and the facts. We need to look past the rhetoric and get to the meat of the issues. In addition, we need to act responsibly as health care consumers by using not abusing the system. We should all be willing to peacefully and respectfully express our ideas, solutions and concerns to those we have elected to represent our interests. You can also have a major impact by having these discussions with your loved ones and the medical professionals you deal with on a regular basis.

Chapter 4

How to Advocate for Someone Else

Advocating for a friend or loved one can be even more challenging than advocating for yourself. There are several circumstances where you may find yourself in a position to advocate for another. Whether it's for a friend, spouse, partner, parent or relative, you may face tough decisions and a laundry list of things to keep track of to insure the desired outcome. Your role may be one of several, such as accompanying someone to an appointment, agreeing to be a Durable Power of Attorney for Health Care or perhaps even to be someone's guardian. Each role comes with different levels of responsibilities. In this chapter we will discuss these roles, their advantages and disadvantages and ways to navigate the healthcare system on someone else's behalf.

You're a good friend
When a friend faces an acute or chronic health condition, he is going to need help and you have decided to be there. What do you do in this role?

Be a good listener
Many times all a friend needs is someone to listen. In this role it is tempting to give advice or, worse yet, share horror stories of other people you know who have had the same problem. Try to fight this temptation. If your friend needs your opinion, he will usually ask.

When he does ask for your opinion it is generally best to resist giving too much direction. If you decide to start telling your friend what he should do and then things don't work out, you are going to be the one catching the blame. If your friend does ask for help in making a health care decision, help him work through the decision making process keeping your personal biases to yourself. Perhaps you can help research a topic, aid in coming up with a list of questions for his care providers or just be another set of ears at appointments.

Be a chauffeur

When a friend is having surgery, chemotherapy, radiation, physical therapy or any type of medical intervention that may interfere with driving abilities, it helps to have someone offer to drive her back and forth. As a chauffeur, let the patient dictate any further assistance she may require. Perhaps she would like you to go in with her, and sometimes she may prefer a little privacy. When assisting a friend by driving to appointments, make sure that you are punctual. Showing up late can cause additional stress to the patient, can result in the loss of the appointment time and can lead to unsafe driving practices. If you have access to more than one car, make sure that you take the car that is most accessible to the patient's physical capabilities. If you do not have a car that can comfortably accommodate the patient's physical abilities, you may suggest that you drive the patient's car or borrow a car from someone else. If a car is not an option, you may want to assist the patient in finding other transportation. Many clinics and health care services will provide transportation at a minimal cost. Your local public transit authority will usually have a service that can accommodate patients who may need special transportation. Finally, if the patient has insurance, encourage the patient to check with her insurance company to see if she has any transportation benefits.

Rally the troops

Sometimes being a friend to someone who has an acute or chronic health issue can become overwhelming for just one person. This is when it is important to recruit help from other friends and family. Spreading the workload can help with everyone's mental health. Most people underestimate the resources in their life that can avail themselves in a time of need. People who are often available to help come from a wide array of groups such as: friends, family, neighbors, support groups, church members, social or professional groups and community associations. These people can assist a patient by fixing meals, pet sitting, house sitting, transportation, house cleaning, errand running or by simply just spending some time visiting to help the patient feel a deeper sense of normalcy. One of our services is writing a letter to friends and family informing them of the types of assistance needed. Perhaps you can design a letter that can be distributed by mail or e-mail. It is often difficult for the patient to ask for help themselves.

The advantages and disadvantages of being a good friend
There are mostly advantages associated with the friendship role. It is an opportunity to give back and to help fill a very important niche in the life of someone who perhaps has been in your life for many years. The disadvantage of being a friend to someone in a health crisis is that it can drastically change the nature and dynamics of the friendship. As long as you, as a friend, respect that your friend is still a viable individual with a need to feel some sense of control and independence all should go well. Keep in mind that there is a difference between helping a friend in need and enabling your friend to do nothing for himself. Part of the healing process or the process of dealing with a progressive illness, is maintaining that sense of independence. It is important to remember to allow the patient to do what he can, when he can. Encouragement and standing back, when appropriate, go a long way in the maintenance of the friendship and the healing process.

Becoming a Durable Power of Attorney for Health Care
This request can come from any number of people including family members, spouses/partners and friends. As someone's Durable Power of Attorney for Health Care, you may be asked to make medical decisions for someone if she should become incapacitated to the point that she no longer has the ability to speak for herself. The Durable Power of Attorney for Health Care designation is different than a Durable Power of Attorney which can involve financial and contractual obligations. When asked to represent someone's health care wishes, make

sure that you have a detailed discussion with that person so that you know exactly what her wishes are. You should also make sure that she has picked a secondary person in case you are unavailable.

As Durable Power of Attorney for Health Care, it will be your responsibility to monitor the health care team's performance, and to ensure that they are doing what the patient desires. You will be the person who the care providers will come to for decisions and the person who they will call when there are changes in the patient's health status. It will also be up to you, when necessary, to keep family and friends updated on any changes in the patient's condition. In the worst case scenario, it may be up to you to make a decision on whether or not to continue life sustaining measures. Make sure that before you take on a role such as this, you have given a great deal of thought to your ability to make the above decisions. If you doubt your abilities to follow through with the decisions, then by all means, inform the person asking you to take on this role. The Durable Power of Attorney for Health Care is perhaps the one role that will allow you to truly advocate for another.

The advantage of being the Durable Power of Attorney for Health Care for someone close to you is that you are being given the opportunity to advocate for someone that you care about. The disadvantages are that it is, at times, a very time consuming responsibility, and you will probably be faced with numerous difficult decisions. The important things to remember are to do your research and to respect the wishes of your loved one.

Become a Guardian
Being a legal guardian for a loved one is a huge responsibility with many associated duties. In the legal guardian role you will not only be responsible for medical decisions and financial matters, but also as a protector, of sorts, for the individual and his rights. A legal guardian is appointed by the court as a result of a request from a family member, hospital, extended care facility or social services agency. You can apply to be the guardian of a friend, neighbor or family member. When applying for guardianship you will be asked to present evidence as

to why the person requires a guardian, and why you are the most qualified to accept the role. If you should apply and be appointed as a guardian for a loved one, keep in mind that most of what you do in this role will be monitored by the courts.

In some cases, a patient may have a legal guardian selected by the court who has no knowledge of the patient's wishes or medical history. This situation is often found when a patient does not have any family or has not thought to appoint someone in advance to act as legal guardian. This is an unfortunate situation, because many times a patient will have very specific wishes in regards to heroic life saving measures which can be ignored when the legal guardian has no direct connection to the patient. To avoid this situation, have these discussions with your loved ones today.

Making health care decisions for another is difficult enough, but when you are not present, it is almost impossible to make decisions that are going to be in the patient's best interest. If, as a legal guardian, you are in a different state from the patient and are unable to be involved in the day-to-day care, you can appoint a Durable Power of Attorney for Health Care who is able to be present in the advocating role. As an advocate in the legal guardian role, stay up to date on the patient's medications, treatments and advance directives. Make sure to keep other family members or interested parties informed. Keeping everyone up to date will increase cohesiveness and cooperation, and will also help to decrease the possibility of suspicions. Once again, when advocating for a patient in the legal guardian role, it is important to be familiar with the patient's wishes regarding his healthcare and end of life decisions.

The advantage of being a legal guardian is that you can help insure that a loved one's care and rights are being protected when he is no longer able to protect himself. It is also a wonderful way to be able to advocate for someone you care about. The disadvantages are, once again, that it is a time consuming process and wrought with tough decisions. The other advantage and/or disadvantage of guardianship can be the fact that the courts are much more involved in this assignment. While it is advantageous that the courts are there to minimize the risk that the patient is being taken advantage of, court involvement can also slow down the process in certain circumstances.

Regardless of the role you find yourself in when dealing with the health care of a loved one, be mindful that there are several things that you need to consider when making health care decisions for someone else.

1. Know the wishes of the patient related to their medical care, medical choices, and also their own definition of quality of life.

2. Keep your personal biases in check.

3. Know the patient's prognosis

4. Know what is or will be the patient's quality of life.

If you find yourself in any one of the above mentioned roles, be mindful of the legal implications of each role. If you have questions, you should consult a trusted legal adviser to discuss your rights and the patient's rights. Each health care facility should also be able to provide you with a copy of the Patients' Bill of Rights.

Chapter 5

Lawyers, Lobbyists, Pharmaceutical and Insurance Companies

The old adage, "you can't live with them and you can't live without them", holds true for lawyers, lobbyists, pharmaceutical and insurance companies. As stated in earlier chapters, health/patient advocacy can take many forms from global to personal. Any way we look at these issues, they affect us all on a personal level. The one way that we can deal with some of these intangible issues is to advocate for ourselves by being aware of how certain things affect our individual health care.

Lawyers
Lawyers can be very useful to the health care consumer. They can advise us in regards to our advance directives and legal concerns surrounding our health care decisions and designations. They can also help protect our financial assets by advising us how to best plan for future, unforeseen circumstances. Lawyers can also help in the system of checks and balances by keeping the health care community account-able to its patients.

Unfortunately, there are cases of gross negligence and malpractice in health care. When negligence is involved, a lawyer can help the patient pursue legal and financial compensation to cover the cost of injuries or loss of life. Lawyers also play an intricate role in keeping pharmaceutical and insurance companies conscientious in their practices where patients are concerned.

Medical negligence is an area that health care consumers need to look at closely and approach responsibly in order to protect the future of affordable health care. It is a fact of life that many, if not most, health care interventions come with associated risks and benefits. Generally the benefits outweigh the risks, but when risks rear their ugly heads people are picking up the phone to call their attorneys to get their share of the pie. As a health care consumer, you need to ask your provider to thoroughly explain those risks and benefits to you so that you can make an informed decision. While it is unfortunate when any of us experience an undesired affect related to our medical treatment, if it is a stated risk and the standards of care were followed, it does not necessarily fall into the categories of malpractice and/or negligence. Often we see patients filing law suits over adverse events that are considered to be known risks. While these law suits may not have any validity in terms of malpractice/negligence, they are often settled to avoid expensive litigation. These events lead to high malpractice rates for medical providers and increased costs to every health care consumer. As you advocate for your own affordable health care, weigh your health care outcomes carefully. If you become a victim of negligence or malpractice, pursue your legal rights. If you suffer an adverse affect from a known risk of an intervention, give careful consideration to your next step in your personal advocacy process.

Being both a health care consumer and a nurse, I have seen how the medical profession has changed because of legal implications. Medical schools are now teaching doctors how to practice to avoid litigation. Many of the newer doctors rely less on their physical assessment skills and more on diagnostic testing. The new developments in diagnostic testing can truly enhance patient safety and diagnosis of disease processes, but when overused or used inappropriately, they can also be harmful and unduly expensive to you, the health care consumer. As an advocate for yourself you can, with the help of your medical provider, decide the risks and benefits of more expensive diagnostic testing, and what other alternatives may be available. As stated above, almost all medical interventions come with their own inherent set of risks. So while doctors are ordering more tests to aid with diagnosis and using more treatment protocols to treat or prevent disease processes, they may be increasing your risks of adverse events. Once again, be informed, be active in your care and have these discussions with your medical providers.

Here are some very common medical interventions and tests and the inherent risks and benefits associated with them.

Antibiotic therapy
Antibiotics are truly a benefit to our society. Prior to antibiotics many people died of bacterial infections. While antibiotic therapy has been credited in saving many lives, it also comes with several risks. Antibiotics can cause severe allergic reactions in some patients. They can also cause secondary infections by destroying the normal flora in the body. In addition, antibiotics may result in some very unpleasant side effects such as nausea, vomiting, diarrhea, headache, etc. Obviously when a serious bacterial infection is involved, the benefits of antibiotic therapy generally outweigh the risks. In recent years, however, there have been an increased number of bacteria that have become resistant to current antibiotic choices. Part of the problem has been that patients go to their doctors requesting antibiotics for viral conditions which are not helped by antibiotics. As an advocate for yourself, talk with your medical provider about the responsible use of antibiotic therapy.

IV therapy and blood draws
These are two very common medical interventions that most of us have had at one time or another.

Both are very useful in medical treatment and diagnosis, but both also come with associated risks. When you puncture the skin there is always a risk of bacteria entering the blood stream which can cause both local and systemic infections. In addition, even when standards of care and good technique are used, there are risks of vein collapse and infiltration. Once again, while both carry risks, they are very useful tools used by your medical provider.

Medications

Both prescription and over-the-counter medications have enhanced many of our lives. They make us feel better, and they treat or cure many disease processes. As useful as medications are, they all come with associated risks. Generally, we find that the benefits outweigh the risks, but once again we can see some very serious complications that arise from their use.

As advocates for our own health care, we need to look at the legal implications when the risks of these interventions present themselves. Do we pursue legal action when we engage in these interventions knowing what the risks are? Are we using the legal system to promote accountability of medical professionals or for personal gain? These are decisions that require responsible thought and the balancing of personal accountability. We, as health advocates for ourselves, need to look at not only the personal impact of our decisions, but also the global impact on our health care system.

Lobbyists

The political lobbying industry has been active throughout the history of the democratic process. In the early days, lobbying was done on a rather informal basis in social settings. The lobbyists would hang out in places where lawmakers socialized, and enter into conversations with the legislators and their staff to promote their groups' interests. The early lobbyists represented small special interest groups and grassroots organizations. Over the years this process has grown expo-nentially. While there are still lobbyists who work with the grassroots organizations and small special interest groups, the profession has expanded to represent entire industries and large groups with special interests.

Understanding how lobbyists and the lobbying industry affect our health care system is a complex procedure. There are many who have tried to study the impact that lobbying has had on our political process, but have found it difficult to measure its exact influence. One thing for sure, there are hundreds of millions of dollars spent every year on lobbying efforts. If the industry was not having an influence on our political process, it is a good bet that the business would not be growing by leaps and bounds. An example of the scope of lobbying is demonstrated by a study conducted by the Center for Public Integrity. This study found that between January of 2005 and June of 2006, the pharmaceutical industry alone spent around 182 million dollars on federal lobbying. If you consider that all major players in our health care system such as insurance companies, hospitals, nursing homes, physician and nursing groups hire lobbyists, you can realize the vast amount of money spent on influencing our legislators.

Part of being your own health advocate is being aware of how both the lobbying industry and our political system work in influencing your personal health care costs and access to the health care system. One question that you may ask yourself is what is this costing me? If health care related industries are spending hundreds of millions of dollars every year on lobbying, how is this influencing our costs of their services? You may also ask if the lobbying industry is an asset or liability in representing your interests related to health care. Regardless of how you answer these questions, as an advocate for yourself or others, you should try to raise your awareness and involve-ment to insure that the services offered by the health care system are there when you need them.

Pharmaceutical Companies
The pharmaceutical industry is very active in the lobbying effort. The industry lobbies for changes in reimbursement, sales, marketing, research, and legislation regarding creation of new drugs and other pharmaceuticals. The industry also lobbies for protection from lawsuits stemming from adverse effects from products they produce. Recently, the pharmaceutical industry has become increasingly active in marketing their products direct to the health care consumer through aggressive advertising campaigns.

What impact do their efforts have on you and your health care? The lobbying can affect the costs of the medications we use to maintain our health or control our disease processes. The other impact can be in the development of new drugs and services that can enhance our lives. Finally, the advertising can make us more knowledgeable health care consumers. That being said, we again need to be active in our approach to an industry that has major influences on our personal health care. While pharmaceutical advertising can be beneficial in increasing our knowledge about what is on the market, the information needs to be put in its proper context. As with any advertising, it requires personal research and scrutiny when applied to our individual health needs. Keep in mind that the goal of advertising is to sell a product, and may not be the best source of unbiased information. In addition to the advertising of their products, pharmaceutical companies also offer programs to financially assist patients in obtaining their products. Some of these programs can be very helpful in defraying some of the expense of the medications, but once again do your research and talk to your medical care provider about whether those products are best suited for your individual medical needs.

Overall, the pharmaceutical industry has played a significant role in extending life expectancy, enhancing our quality of life and influencing our health care decisions. As health care consumers and advocates we should, once again, approach our use of the pharmaceutical products responsibly. We can do this by paying attention to the industry's lobbying efforts and their influence on us as individuals. We can also be savvy when it comes to the advertising of pharmaceuticals by knowing not only the benefits, but the associated risks. These activities involve researching and engaging our health care providers in discussions regarding the responsible use of the products on the market.

Health Insurance Companies

Insurance companies play a big role in the health care industry and have been a part of the ever-changing evolution of health care services. As with any insurance product, health insurance companies operate on the basis of calculated risks and profit margins. As health care reform evolves, so will health insurance as we know it. The health insurance industry also participates heavily in lobbying to ensure that their interests are represented and protected.

Advocating for yourself involves monitoring these lobbying actions, and studying the impact that they will have on you and your family. While it may seem like a daunting task to keep track of lobbying activities and legislation regarding health insurance concerns, each individual can make an impact through the election process, where you spend your health care dollars, writing letters to your political representatives and being an informed consumer.

The other part of being an informed consumer is to watch the expenses that your insurance company is or is not paying on your behalf. This also applies if you or a loved one is covered by Medicaid and/or Medicare. All of us need to pay attention to the Explanation of Benefits. Medicare fraud is a huge business and is becoming a very profitable crime. Criminals are accessing and billing the Medicare system for billions of dollars in fraudulent claims every year. This crime is not only a result of poor oversight by our federal government, but also of apathy by health care consumers who do not monitor the expenses billed on their behalf. Many health care consumers give their medical provider their insurance card, pay the co-pay or deductible if applicable, receive an Explanation of Benefits and pay any additional amounts that are billed without thinking. Although consumers are not happy to shell out additional monies, they will because they believe that there is nothing else that they can do. In fact, there are several things that you can do that will not only lower your own costs, but also the overall costs of health care.

The first thing that you can do is to know your policy and your coverage. If you don't feel like reading through a thick coverage manual, then call your health insurance company to see if your planned testing or treatment is covered. Occasionally, health insurance companies will pay completely for one type of test that has been an industry standard for several years, but will not pay for a newer test. Talk with your health care provider to determine if the newer test is most beneficial for you considering your medical history and financial considerations. Secondly, ask for a detailed itemized bill from your health care provider to ensure that what was billed to the insurance company was actually what you received. There are times when your bill will be coded wrong by your care provider, and the insurance company will be paying an expense on your behalf for a test or treatment you did not receive. Thirdly, negotiate with your insurance company when you feel its payment is not in line with what its coverage is supposed to be. An example of this, is when you have a preauthorized surgery. During the surgery there is blood drawn. The blood is sent to the lab for testing, and the results may have an impact on your treatment during the surgery. You get home to find your insurance company did not pay for the lab work, because the hospital's lab was not covered by your insurance plan. While it sounds absurd that they would approve a surgery that most likely will require blood work to be done, yet expect the hospital to send the blood across town to be tested while you are under the gas, it has happened on more than one occasion. This is usually a cost that can be negotiated with the insurance company. It may take some patience, persistence and working your way up the managerial chain, but you can probably convince the health insurance company to pay the bill.

In order to continue to have access to health care, health insurance and affordable coverage, we all need to participate in the process. We need to be responsible for maintaining our own costs and keeping the entities addressed in this chapter accountable. In 2008 alone, the Medicaid Fraud Control Unit recovered 1.3 billion dollars in billing fraud. Keep in mind; this is just what they recovered, not the total amount of fraudulent billing committed. We have also heard about pharmaceutical companies paying doctors to promote and prescribe their products, and recently the FDA admitted to being unduly influenced by legislators who had received lobbying dollars from pharmaceutical companies. Unless each of us takes some personal responsibility in advocating for ourselves in these matters, our health care system will continue to struggle financially. A struggling health care system does not bode well for our individual health care costs, safety and accessibility to the system.

Chapter 6

Health Maintenance

The easiest way to be your own Health Advocate is, of course, to stay healthy and lower your exposure to the health care system. In this chapter, we will discuss some ways to maintain your health and how to use the health care system to your benefit. Some of the points in this chapter will seem like common sense, but they are issues that we see in the health care system on a daily basis. Over the course of the next few pages, we will discuss lifestyle choices, preventative activities and health maintenance activities.

Let's start our discussion with the topics that we read about every day, eating right, exercise and elimination of bad habits.

Eating Right
The good news is that we are not going to give you a specific diet to follow, but instead provide some ideas on how to incorporate healthy eating and dietary changes into your life without it becoming all consuming. I think that it is safe to say that we all have probably at one point been on a diet, thought about being on a diet and/or bought the latest book on how to lose weight and then we have gone back to where we find comfort and ease. Hopefully, you will find the following suggestions easy to follow and easy to incorporate into your daily lifestyle while not increasing your stress level.

Going on a diet is usually a recipe for failure. Once you have eliminated any chance of metabolic disorders that could be affecting your weight maintenance, it generally boils down to calories in and calories out. Weighing food and looking up calorie counts can indeed be a time consuming process. The good news is, we typically eat a lot of the same foods on a daily or weekly basis. Whether it is the routine breakfast, favorite comfort foods or dining at our favorite eating establishments, our food choices tend to be rather predictable. The benefit to our predictability is that it makes keeping track of calories a little easier. Once you get use to recognizing portion sizes and have looked up your foods for a week or two, you can get a pretty close estimation of your daily caloric intake without the measuring and looking up of calories every time. The internet is also a good resource for general calorie counting and provides nutritional information for many restaurants and fast food chains.

The first key is to make the changes that you can maintain without feeling like a failure. The drawback to most diets is that they are a drastic change from our norm and difficult to maintain. When we go on a diet and stray from the regime, we view ourselves as failing which sets up a pattern of self-criticism and overeating as a compensatory mechanism. If you can gradually make changes that can become a permanent part of your lifestyle and give yourself a failure without guilt once in a while, you will no doubt start seeing some positive results in obtaining a better weight control pattern.

Eating out does not have to be a recipe for disaster.
While most restaurants offer portion sizes that are generally way bigger than we need or should be eating, it is possible to work toward weight maintenance without giving up what has become a social outlet for many of us. Many restaurants offer senior portions or half portions. It is also possible to split a meal with your dining companion. By cutting down on portion sizes and working toward better choices, you can still enjoy eating out without sabotaging weight maintenance. For myself, I found that when eating out I very much underestimated the calorie values for some of my favorite foods. With the knowledge garnered from many of the restaurants' websites, I was able to make better choices without too much denying.

Eat your way up the food pyramid.
If you look at the food pyramid and work your way up, it is obvious
that the biggest portion of the pyramid includes the fruits and vegetables and the smallest part is the dairy and meats. If you start at the
bottom of the pyramid getting the servings of fruits and vegetables in
as the day progresses, by the time you get to the smallest portion of
the pyramid you don't have a lot of room left for the foods that are not
as good for you. The result is that you now have consumed more food,
less calories and healthier overall choices.

**Make meal preparation an artistic creation and/or a social
outlet.** Instead of looking at healthy meal preparation as a chore
and time consuming project, make it fun and involve your family and
friends. The fact is that a huge part of our interactions with friends
and family center around eating. Instead of always meeting at your
favorite restaurant, plan meals at home having everyone contribute.
Create meal ideas ahead of time when you have some downtime on
weekends and evenings. Planning early and shopping ahead will make
the process easier to fit into your busy lifestyle. The other advantage
of preparing more of your own meals is that you have greater control
and knowledge of the calorie content of your meal.

Know your weaknesses and how your mind works.
As an example, back in my dieting days I would clear out my
cupboards of all my favorite snack food and then start with the latest
diet plan. The problem this created was all I could do was think about
what I was missing. Consequently, I would find myself going out and
buying a bag of my favorite chocolates, and eating the whole thing at
once so that I could start the diet process again. Needless to say this
plan did not work too well. What it took decades to realize was that I
personally did better when I kept my favorite chocolates in the house
avoiding the binging cycle. I found the key was to exercise some self
restraint: put the chocolate where it is more challenging to get and
just take one and put the rest back. With this method, if I wanted
more I had to go dig them out of the hiding spot. Most times I decided
it was not worth the effort. Consequently, I stopped obsessing about
what I did not have; I stopped the binging cycle and was able to satisfy

my sweet tooth without wrecking what was otherwise a pretty good eating plan.

Get creative with your social life. As discussed earlier, eating has become the center of many of our social and family relationships. Dining with the family allows us to discuss the day's activities and keep in touch with what is going on in the lives of those close to us. We also use eating as an excuse to get together with friends and have a little escape time. While we can use these opportunities to plan healthful meals and experiment with healthier eating, that rarely occurs. So if we cannot use food as a social outlet and maintain a reasonable nutrition plan, then we need to come up with some alternative activities to accomplish the same goals. Pick an activity that everyone enjoys that does not involve food. Think of alternatives that will allow you to catch up with the family and escape with friends. Taking short walks, playing games, going to parks and zoos are just a few of the activities that can take the place of eating as the center of social activities.

Exercising

Once again, we are going to address some common sense approaches in this section. Some people like to incorporate exercise into their daily routines and others find it a struggle just to get off the couch. Exercise can help to either minimize your exposure to the health care system or put you right into the center of it all. A regular exercise program can help boost your immune system and enhance your heart, lungs and circulatory systems. Too much exercise or a too aggressive workout program can lower your immunity and result in injury and chronic musculoskeletal problems. Some sensible approaches will help to insure that you minimize your exposure to the health care system.

Start slow. If you are not already accustomed to daily exercise, then you need to start out slowly. Don't try to attempt an aggressive exercise program right out of the gate. Starting too aggressively will generally result in injury and failure. If you have never been inclined to exercise, and are thinking of starting a plan, you should consider seeing your doctor to make sure that you don't have any health issues that will be exacerbated by a new exercise program. If you have a known preexisting medical condition such as high blood pressure, heart disease, diabetes or asthma, then you should consult with your health care provider for recommendations on the best type of program for you. If you have exercised in the past, but gave it up, don't expect to pick up where you left off. Start off slowly again and build your way up.

Set realistic goals. Generally when we start an exercise program we have lofty goals. We start out by saying that we are going to work out every day and lose five pounds a week. Once again, we are setting ourselves up for failure. Start with a few minutes a day three or five times a week and gradually build up your time and your days. If you start out slowly and make it a habit that you can easily fit into your busy schedule, you are more likely to maintain it on a regular basis.

Keep it simple. You do not need a gym membership or a lot of expensive equipment to get a decent workout or to maintain a regular workout schedule. A walking program is a good way to get started. You can also incorporate strength, balance and flexibility training into your daily activities. Some easy ideas include balancing on one leg while waiting in line, push-ups on the counter while waiting for the coffee to brew, stretching and resistance bands while sitting at the office or on the couch.

Dietary and Herbal Supplements

Eating a well balanced diet usually provides us with the nutrition needed for good health, but occasionally we need a little boost if we do not maintain the proper balance. When contemplating dietary supplements, make sure that you do some research about the risks and benefits involved. Many people believe if they are taking a supplement that is "natural", there are no adverse side effects. Many dietary and herbal supplements have some very serious side effects, and many also may negatively interact with prescription medications. Before starting a new dietary supplement, check with your family physician, pharmacist, and library and internet research services. Keep in mind that you should also examine the source of the information, to make sure that it is unbiased and not promoting and/or profiting from the information provided. This applies to family physicians as well. While we would like to think that our personal physicians are prescribing medications based only on what is in our best interest, there are times when physicians will have contracts with pharmaceutical companies to promote their brands. Below we will look at some of the more common supplements.

Multivitamins are generally a good all-around supplement, but if you eat a well balanced diet a multivitamin is generally not necessary. There are very few side effects to multivitamins, but if you are taking other supplements or vitamins you should become familiar with the recommended dosages of daily vitamins to ensure that you are not getting too much of a good thing.

Vitamins A, D, E and K are fat soluble vitamins. Because fat soluble vitamins are stored in the fat cells of the body, it is possible to develop a toxic level of these vitamins. If you are taking a multivitamin and one of these fat soluble vitamins, take note of the maximum recommended daily dosages. Vitamin D for example is touted for a number of benefits including prevention of osteoporosis, boosting immunity and cancer prevention. In dosages that exceed the maximum recommendations, Vitamin D can cause serious heart irregularities. Vitamin K is another vitamin that people take to prevent osteoporosis. Vitamin K is generally found in our diets in dark green and leafy vegetables. Vitamin K is stored in the body's fatty tissue and released through the urine when the body does not use it. Vitamin K is also very important in blood clotting. Too much vitamin K can lead to increased risk of blood clots, too little vitamin K can lead to an increased risk of bleeding. If you are taking a blood thinning medication prescribed by your doctor, vitamin K can inhibit the action of these blood thinning medications. If you are taking any of these vitamins in large doses, keep in mind that when levels are too high they will be stored in the liver possibly leading to liver damage. Keep your health care provider informed of your supplementations, and have the levels monitored to ensure that you remain within the recommended guidelines.

Herbal Supplements are plentiful and touted to treat a variety of symptoms and diseases. The main caution related to herbal supplements, is that they are not closely regulated for quality in this country and it is a buyer-beware type of market. Because of the lack of oversight and regulation, there are unfortunately some herbal supplement manufacturers that fail to produce what they say. Do your research before buying these and stay with the proven manufacturers. Once again, just because it says natural, it does not mean that it is beneficial or safe. Check with your health care provider before starting an herbal supplement, and make sure that you list these supplements as part of your medication history when visiting your physician, hospital and/or surgeon.

Two of my favorite dietary supplements are garlic and apple cider vinegar with the Mother (the sediment). Both have been touted to lower cholesterol levels and blood pressure. Vinegar has also been touted over the centuries to boost immunity, improve joint health, purify the urinary and gastrointestinal tracts and treat a wide array of viruses and injuries. While both of these supplementations have been around for ages and are relatively safe and beneficial, it is still important to consult with your health care provider before beginning. Garlic, for example, is known to thin blood. If you are taking aspirin and/or blood thinners and start a garlic supplement, the consequences can be very dangerous. In addition, because both supplements have been shown to have an effect on blood pressure and cholesterol, if you are taking medications to lower your blood pressure and cholesterol, your levels could become too low. If you would rather start a natural supplement to attempt to maintain healthy levels, discuss the risks and benefits with your health care provider.

If your doctor is concerned that you are developing early onset high blood pressure, high cholesterol and/or borderline diabetes, you can talk with your health care provider about trying natural remedies before progressing to prescription medications. Many physicians now are open to discussing non-pharmacological treatments for early and borderline disease processes. With lifestyle modifications and natural remedies, you can sometimes turn borderline conditions around, but make sure that you do this in conjunction with medical supervision and not on your own. While catching and treating these conditions early can decrease your risk of more severe health issues, ignoring them and failing to monitor your progress can lead to serious life-threatening conditions.

Maintaining a balanced life

Perhaps the best to way to maintain your health and avoid the health care system as much as possible is to maintain a balanced lifestyle. This, as with many things in life, is easier said than done. Here are just a few suggestions that may serve as a reminder or guide to help you strike a balance in your life.

1. All work and no play…We have all heard this little ditty and there is probably a good reason for its popularity. Too much work affects our lives in many ways. Long hours at work decrease sleep time, decrease time for recreation and fitness activities, increase stress levels, and increase our chances of running down our immunity; all of which increase our chances of acute and chronic illnesses. When deciding what the right amount of work is, we need to look at several factors. Are you working too much because it is required to make the minimum needed to sustain life or to sustain your lifestyle? Or, are you working more than expected to avoid dealing with other issues in your life? Or, perhaps you are working to sustain someone else's lifestyle? These are just a few of the factors that can cause an imbalance in many people's lives.

If your work life is out of balance, it is just a matter of time before your health is affected. Take steps to try get the balance back by looking at your lifestyle, dealing with issues that are driving you to work too much, and looking at those around you who may be draining you either financially and/or emotionally. These are major changes and will take time, patience and diligence. The more work that you put into these issues the more quickly you will strike a healthier balance in your life and avoid the health pitfalls that often accompany these imbalances.

2. Sleep is the body's way of healing and restoring itself and is yet another important factor in avoiding the health care system and maintaining your health. The gold standard has always been at least eight hours a night for adults, but very few adults get that amount of sleep in any given night. Whether or not everyone functions best on eight hours of sleep is still up for debate. I am sure that you know someone who tells you that she does great on only four or five hours a night. Perhaps those people can make it through most days without incident, but is this person you want flying your plane, operating on you or sharing the road with you.

The fact is, we need to plan a good seven to eight hours for good restorative sleep per day. As with most aspects of life, natural sleep is better, but if you find this challenging, there are natural substances that you can take to aid in getting to sleep. There are also many products on the market that contain alcohol and Diphenhydramine to help induce sleep. While these methods may assist you in getting to sleep, they often interfere with the natural sleep cycle and after a while the body builds up a tolerance to them making them less effective. Prescription sleep aids also have the same drawbacks and require a thorough conversation with your health care provider. Many of the prescription sleep aids are addictive and require higher and higher dosages to be effective. The one time when prescription sleep aids may be beneficial, is after a traumatic event that leads to increased anxiety and sleep disorders. Once again, a conversation with your health care provider should take place to insure the best results. Any sleep aid should be used only on a short term basis to try to re-establish a normal sleep cycle. Caution must also be taken when there is a history of severe depression and/or suicidal ideation. In these cases, it is important to make sure that there is someone available to insure compliance and guard against abuse and overdose.

To help develop a regular, restorative sleep pattern, treat sleep like you would many other aspects of your life, put it in your schedule. A regularly scheduled sleep pattern helps the body follow its natural cycles and will provide you with stronger immunity, better weight control, greater concentration abilities and an overall healthier lifestyle.

3. De-cluttering your life is another way to achieve balance. There have been many studies that show that people who have a lot of clutter in their lives suffer from increased anxiety and stress, less ability to concentrate and more health problems. Clutter can come in many forms such as a cluttered living environment, a cluttered calendar, a cluttered financial picture and/or a cluttered emotional state. Generally, if you have clutter in one area of your life, you have clutter issues in most, if not all areas. Getting the clutter out of your life takes diligence, patience, determination and motivation.

As with the other things we have discussed in this chapter, start with one area and daily work your way up to where you want to be. If you have a cluttered environment, start with one corner in one room. Decide what you want to keep, donate, give away or sell, and then do it. Move to the next area until the clutter is gone. Clutter creates stress, decreases productivity and often leads to, or is derived from, a depressive state or an avoidance of a bigger issue in your life. Examine these issues as you go to avoid falling into the same trap in the future. The physical clutter in your environment is generally reflective of an imbalance in another area of your life. Starting with your physical environment helps you to identify the imbalances in the other areas. Perhaps the clutter is a result of excessive spending, which leads to an increased need for income, leading to working more to pay for the increased spending.

As you work on the de-cluttering and the uncovering of the reasons for it, remind yourself of what is important in your life. Are you one who likes to buy a lot of toys and distractions, just to find out that you have to spend more time working to pay for them and have no time to play with them? Simplifying your life will, in the long run, lead to better health maintenance.

Elimination of bad habits
Eliminating bad habits in our life can be most challenging. Whether it is overeating, smoking, alcohol/drug abuse or inactivity, we need to approach a bad habit, once again, with diligence and with an eye toward what is motivating our decisions to participate in these choices.

1. Smoking cessation is one of the most challenging undertakings. The addictive nature of nicotine has been compared to that of heroin and cocaine. There are many non-smoking aids on the market, both prescription and over-the-counter, each having its own advantages and disadvantages. Before picking a stop smoking method, consider what the best way for you is and have a discussion with your health care provider.

   The first way to stop smoking is the natural way by going cold turkey and modifying your behavior. Behavior modification takes self-discipline and finding ways to distract yourself from the act of smoking. Thanks to non-smoking laws and increased taxation, the government has given you a head start on modifying your behavior. The inability to smoke in most public places is the first step in the modification of behavior, and with the increased cost of tobacco products, the cost for many has become prohibitive.

   Many smokers have either an oral fixation or a hand to mouth tendency. These aspects are why many smokers who contemplate quitting fear weight gain. This is a valid concern and many smokers who quit do experience at least some initial weight gain. To combat this problem, try sugar-free gums and candies. You can also try holding something in your hand such as a straw to satisfy the need of having something to do with your hands besides smoking. Increasing your exercise and water intake is also helpful in flushing the nicotine out of your system. If this is the method you choose to quit smoking, additional help and support can be had by finding a support group or contacting one of the many quit smoking hotlines that can be found online at www.smokefree.gov. Some other tips that can help you successfully break your smoking habit are:

   1. Set a day to quit and tell everyone you know when the day is.

   2. Get rid of all of your tobacco products and accessories such as ashtrays, lighters and matches.

3. Start a journal to track your cravings and emotions.

4. Have an ample supply of sugar-free gums and candies.

5. Carry a list of websites and phone numbers that you can contact for support and encouragement.

6. Avoid triggers to smoking such as drinking alcohol and overeating.

7. Increase your water intake. Put your water into a bottle or glass with a straw to satisfy the urge of inhaling.

8. Get plenty of rest to avoid feeling tired and needing that energy boost provided by nicotine.

9. Take it one day at a time, and if you backslide, start again. Each time you quit the easier it gets. Don't get discouraged if it does not take the first time.

If the above method does not appeal to you or has not worked, you may want to try some of the over-the-counter aides such as nicotine gums, lozenges, patches or the smokeless cigarettes. Most of these aides come in different doses of nicotine depending on your amount of tobacco use. While these aides help in decreasing the cravings, they do not do much for the hand-to-mouth habit. Because nicotine based aides contain the same components as stimulants, it will take longer to see and feel the total benefits of smoking cessation. The advantage is that they do not contain the tar and other additives found in the tobacco-based products. When taking the nicotine aides, follow the package recommendations on dosages. Nicotine will contribute to increased blood pressure and will continue to put a stress on your cardiovascular and circulatory systems.

The third method of smoking cessation is to visit your health
care provider and a get a prescription for one of the medications
designed to help the mind and body break the addiction. These
drugs work on the neurotransmitters in the brain. While these
medications don't contain any tar, nicotine or other additives found
in tobacco products, they do come with a long list of side effects.
Even though these drugs are available by prescription and have
been approved by the FDA, it is important to discuss the risks and
benefits with your health care provider.

2. Alcohol and substance abuse are two more areas of addiction that
   can take a huge toll on your health maintenance. There are many
   levels of use and abuse, and the root causes of such addictions are
   often complex and generally require a multidisciplinary approach
   to combat.

Light social drinking has been credited with some health benefits and
is generally not a problem in maintaining a healthy lifestyle. While
there are some health benefits to moderate alcohol consumption, care
needs to be taken when taking medications including over-the-counter
medications.

When alcohol consumption becomes a problem, it can have a huge
impact on most if not all aspects of a drinker's life. The health problems are magnified by the stress and issues created in jobs, relationships and financial areas. There are varying degrees of alcoholism
from the functional alcoholic to the alcoholic that can no longer maintain even the basic aspects of life. Regardless of the degree, the health
effects can be drastic and long term. The treatment of alcoholism
should be a multi-disciplinary approach that involves medical maintenance as well as psychological involvement to get to the root of the
disease.

The same method of treatment applies to substance abuse. As with
alcohol abuse, substance abuse can take many forms from the abuse of
street drugs to over-the-counter and prescriptions drugs.

Many times substance abuse starts as a social outlet and then becomes a crutch and addiction. Regardless of the source, street or prescription, the health impact can once again be monumental.

To get help with any addiction, start with an honest conversation with your health care provider. Keep in mind that health care providers are there to help not report you to law enforcement. If your health care provider is part of the problem, writing prescriptions without awareness of a developing problem, then it is usually best to switch providers or utilize one of the many community groups that are available to help with addictions. To determine whether you or a loved one is developing an addiction problem to alcohol, drugs or food start by answering several questions:

1. Is your reliance on food, drugs or alcohol controlling your actions?

2. Are you hiding your use from friends and relatives and/or using alone?

3. Is the use of the substance creating problems in your social, work, financial or family life?

4. Do you go to bed and wake up thinking about the object of abuse?

5. Are you experiencing health problems caused by the addiction?

6. Are you giving up other favorite activities?

7. Are family members and friends questioning you about your use?

Health Maintenance Screenings

Screenings are another important part of good health maintenance.
Screenings are getting a lot of publicity and will no doubt continue
to be in the headlines as health care reform continues to progress.
Regardless of health care reform, health screenings will always be
debated by experts in the field. So what are you to do and who are you
to believe? The best advice is to stay up to date on the latest recommendations, have the appropriate discussions with your health care
provider and consider your own personal feelings and family medical
history. Below we will discuss some of the screening tools available
and the advantages, disadvantages and treatment options currently
available.

Mammography

Mammography recommendations have been in the news a lot lately
and are ones that even many experts can't agree on. The traditional
beliefs were that women should have their first, baseline mammogram
by the age of 35 and then every year after age 40 up to age 80. The
new guidelines are recommending mammography every two years
between the ages of 50 and 74 years. So why the changes?

The changes are based on various studies on the topic. The studies
looked at the number of breast cancer cases diagnosed throughout
the life span, the risk of repeated radiation exposure over time, the
number of both false positive and false negative test results, and the
number of procedures performed to get a more definitive diagnosis.
Some of these studies also focused on the costs associated with the
above mentioned items. While none of us like to put a price tag on
our health, the fact is that part of being a responsible health care
consumer is to look at the costs versus the risks and benefits and to
use this information to make informed decisions for ourselves and our
families. Let's examine some of the known facts about breast cancer
and breast cancer screening.

The risk of breast cancer increases with age, with the majority of
cancers occurring between the ages of 50 and 74 years old. The fact
is, all of us have probably known or knows of someone younger than

50 who has been diagnosed with breast cancer. Besides age, there are other things that can influence the risk and development of breast cancer. Genetic predisposition/family history is a huge predictor for breast cancer especially early onset breast cancer. While there is not much that you can do about the genetic present that your parents gave you on your birthday, there are life style choices that also impact the risk and development of breast cancer. Smoking, obesity, diet and lack of exercise are just a few things that can increase the risk of breast cancer.

So what recommendations should you follow? Once again, have a discussion with your health care providers, know your risk factors, know the risks and benefits from mammography and then formulate your answers. Certainly, if you have a strong family history of breast cancer, you may want to consider starting mammography at an earlier age, and try to lower the risk factors that you have control over. If you do not have a strong family history, you may want to wait and follow the newer guidelines. If you should notice any changes in the look or feel of your breasts, any nipple changes or discharge or find any lumps, make an appointment with your health care provider to have it checked out and discuss the risks and benefits of a mammogram.

The new recommended guidelines also question the benefits of breast self-exam. They feel that women are either not finding problems themselves or that they are finding things that are not indicative of a problem. There are many changes in the breast tissue that are benign and are often related to a woman's menstrual cycle. Nonetheless, the predominate opinion in health care is, it is better to be aware of your body and take notice of changes in order to catch disease processes in their early stages. If there are benign changes, it is better to know that than to ignore something that may be of a more serious nature, or worse yet increase your stress level by worrying about something versus getting your questions answered.

Prostate Screening

This is another area where there is some current debate being generated for many of the same reasons as mammography: the risks and
benefits of early screening versus the costs and unnecessary procedures being generated by false positive screenings.

There are a couple of tests that are traditionally used to screen for
prostate cancer: the digital rectal exam and the prostate specific
antigen (PSA) blood test. The digital rectal exam is performed by a
health care provider and can determine if the prostate is enlarged. An
enlarged prostate is not necessarily indicative of cancer. It is estimated that 50 percent of men over 50 have enlarged prostates. The
PSA blood test where levels are high is more predictive of prostate
cancer, but not always definitive.

The decision when to start screening for prostate cancer should again
be decided after a discussion with your health care provider. The
current school of thought is, if you have a strong family history of
prostate cancer, you may want to discuss screenings with your doctor
at the age of 40. Most other men can wait until 50 to have this discussion. If your family history is positive for early onset prostate cancer,
then you may want to talk with your health care provider about
starting the digital rectal exams even earlier or at the first signs of
any problems or enlargements in the prostate gland.

As stated earlier, many men suffer from an enlarged prostate that
is not cancerous, but nonetheless can cause some very disconcerting
symptoms such as urinary frequency and retention. Certainly if you
experience these symptoms, you should consult your health care
provider for the proper screenings and treatments. There are several
medicines on the market to treat the enlargement as well as surgical
interventions that can be undertaken when the symptoms are more
severe or not responsive to the pharmacological methods.

Cervical Cancer Screenings

Cervical cancer screening is accomplished through Pap smears. The current recommendations state that Pap smears should begin three years after women become sexually active or by 21 years of age. There are two types of Pap smears available. The original smear which has been around for years is the less expensive one and not as sensitive as the newer liquid based smear.

If you and your doctor decide on the least expensive test, which most insurance companies will pay for in full, the recommendation is to have a Pap smear every year. If you decide on the liquid based test, which most insurance companies will pay a portion of, then you can go every two years. If by age 30 you have had three normal Pap tests in a row, the recommendations are for a repeat test every 2 or 3 years. After age 70, with 3 normal Pap smears and no abnormal Pap smears in the last ten years, you may want to discuss stopping the screenings with your health care provider. If you should have any risk factors such as a weakened immune system or HIV infection, then you should talk to your provider about the risks and benefits of continued screenings.

Colon/Rectal Cancer Screenings

The industry standards for Colon/Rectal screenings for both men and women recommend baseline screenings starting at age 50. Once again, with a strong family history of cancer or early onset cancer you may want to discuss starting at an earlier age with your health care provider. Also, if you have a history of any inflammatory bowel disease, colitis or Chron's disease, you may want to discuss earlier screenings as these conditions can increase the risk for cancer development.

There are several ways to test for colorectal cancer. There are tests that can be done on the stool that test for blood and/or DNA predictors of cancer. These tests are fairly reliable as preliminary testing, but may miss certain types of colorectal cancers. The other tests such as colonoscopy, flexible sigmoidoscopy and CT colonoscopy are generally more definitive. Once again, a thorough knowledge of the risks and benefits, and conversations with your health care providers should take place before deciding which screening is going to be best for you.

Ovarian/Uterine/Endometrial Cancer Screenings

These cancers are more difficult and generally more invasive to test for. If you have a family history or experience unexpected or irregular bleeding, it is advisable to speak with your health care provider about undertaking these investigations. There are several screening techniques being investigated that may soon make screening for these cancers more predictive. Stay informed and alert to changes in your body. Ovarian cancer, for example, has very subtle symptoms and many people don't experience overt symptoms until the cancer has become fairly advanced. Be alert for subtle changes in the amount of bloating, urinary frequency, lower abdominal pain and back pain that you are experiencing, as they can be some of the early signs.

Skin Cancer Screenings

These screenings should begin very early in life. Most family doctors and pediatricians can do initial skin assessments. For questionable spots, a dermatologist is the best bet. While sunshine is an important ingredient to good health providing vitamin D and mood elevation, it can also be very damaging to the skin. It only takes about 15 minutes of sunshine a day to provide the necessary vitamin D for most people. Extended, unprotected sun exposure can be quite damaging not only to the skin, but also individual health. With the increased prevalence of tanning beds and sun worshipping, there has been a proportionate rise in skin cancer cases.

To reduce your risks of skin cancer, protect your skin with a high quality sunscreen with both UVA and UVB protection, avoid tanning beds and stay covered during peak sun times. Keep in mind, the sun's rays can penetrate clothing so even areas that are covered are getting at least some exposure. If you discover any sores that won't heal, irregular looking moles and /or skin discolorations, see your health care provider for a thorough skin assessment.

Oral Cancer Screenings

Visiting your dentist on a regular basis is another important aspect of health maintenance. Everyone should have periodic oral cancer screenings. These screenings are even more important for tobacco users and people with a family history of oral cancers.

Blood Pressure Screenings

High blood pressure (hypertension) is often called the silent killer because often the signs and symptoms are not obvious and go undetected for years, slowly damaging the circulatory, cardiac and other major organ systems of the body. Having your blood pressure checked on a regular basis can catch the disease in its earliest stages. If you find your blood pressure consistently creeping up, you can take steps to reverse the trend through life style choices.

Many cases of early onset hypertension can be reversed through increased exercise, smoking cessation, diet control and stress reduction. There are some natural dietary supplements that have shown some success in lowering borderline hypertension such as garlic and apple cider vinegar with the Mother. Talk with your health care provider about the possibilities. When possible it is better to control things naturally rather than starting on prescription medications.

You can monitor your blood pressure yourself at home, but there are some considerations to keep in mind when doing this. Purchase a quality, reliable blood pressure monitoring system. You can check with your local pharmacist or health care provider to choose the one that is right for you. The device should fit properly, be user friendly and accurate. It is best to take your blood pressure at the same time of day and generally just once a week. If you are experiencing symptoms of increased blood pressure such as headaches, blurred vision, nose bleeds, skin flushing and anxiety, you can take your pressure more frequently. Keep in mind that you should not sit in front of your machine taking your blood pressure over and over again. The more times that you take your blood pressure at one sitting the more inaccurate readings become for two reasons. First, it takes a while for the vessels to return to their normal state. Second, the longer you sit there worrying about your blood pressure, the higher your pressure will go.

If you record three consistently high readings over a period of several weeks, you should consult with your health care provider to discuss lifestyle changes or a possible medication regime. A normal blood pressure reading is 120/80. Borderline high readings generally run around 140/90 with high readings considered to be above 140/90. If your top number exceeds 200 and the bottom number exceeds 100, you should consult with health care provider in a timely manner. If your numbers get that high and you are experiencing the above mentioned symptoms, you may want to consider a visit to your family doctor, urgent care or emergency room.

Blood pressure can also run below the average numbers of 120/80. Many people, who exercise regularly, are near their ideal body weight and make healthy lifestyle choices may find their blood pressure to be much lower than normal. Generally, this is no cause for concern. If you experience symptoms of low blood pressure such as extreme fatigue, headaches, dizziness or lightheadedness, you should consult your health care provider.

Diabetes Screening
Diabetes or high blood sugar is another one of those silent killers that can be ravaging your body without any early signs or symptoms. This is why it is important to periodically have your blood sugar levels checked as part of an annual physical or during a health fair opportunity. If you are experiencing any signs or symptoms of diabetes such as increased thirst, increased urination and/or prolonged healing of sores, you should make an appointment with your health care provider to have those levels checked.

Cholesterol Screening
High cholesterol levels can be either genetic and/or lifestyle related. Either way, regular screenings should be done. Even if you have a genetic predisposition for high cholesterol, lifestyle choices can impact your levels. Decreasing fat intake, increasing fiber intake and exercise will help. Once again, it is better to control these levels naturally, but if you have done everything possible to keep your levels down and they

remain high, then you may want to have a conversation with your health care provider about pharmaceutical methods of lowering your levels.

Health Maintenance and disease prevention are also achieved through a thorough vaccination program that starts in childhood and continues into and through adulthood. As with seemingly everything in health care, there have been controversies surrounding vaccines. Over the years there have been concerns about childhood vaccines causing Autism and various neurological disorders. For the most part, the risks of vaccines have been outweighed by the benefits, and the elimination of many catastrophic diseases such as polio, small pox and other diseases that have devastated many cultures throughout history. In this section, we will review some of the vaccines and schedules that have been promoted to help in health maintenance and disease prevention.

Childhood Vaccines
The childhood vaccine schedule is complex and is updated on a regular basis based on current trends and research. The best source for the list of vaccines and schedules is the Centers for Disease Control website at http://www.cdc.gov/. Childhood vaccines may begin in the hospital before discharge home. The vaccines should then be continued through adolescence and early adulthood by the child's pediatrician. As a parent, it is important to keep an accurate record of vaccines. Most health care providers will provide you with a booklet to track the vaccination record. It is important to take this record with you and have it updated as needed.

While most childhood vaccines have been around for years and the safety and efficacy of the vaccines has been proven, there are some new vaccines on the market that are causing a little more controversy and certainly ones that you may want to discuss with your health care provider.

The newest childhood vaccine being recommended is the HPV vaccine that protects against the Human Papillomavirus. HPV is a virus that is spread through sexual contact and can result in the contraction of genital warts as well as cancers of the vagina, vulva and cervix. The vaccine thus far has demonstrated a high degree of safety, but is still being tracked related to its newness on the market. Some of the controversy surrounding this vaccine is that per 100,000 persons vaccinated, the rate of adverse reactions runs fractionally higher than the deaths caused by cervical cancer. The other main controversy is the cost versus the benefit of the vaccine. While this vaccine is mostly being given to adolescent girls, young boys are now starting to receive the vaccine in the hopes that the spread of disease is decreased via that method as well. The vaccine is being given as early as 11 years of age before children become sexually active.

As stated, HPV is a sexually transmitted virus. In most people there are no signs or symptoms of HPV, and generally the virus will go away on its own without treatment. The problem is that while one is infected with the virus, spreading it is quite possible and most likely probable. Even though HPV can go away without treatment, it does cause an increased risk of the above mentioned viruses and cancers.

When deciding whether you or your child should be vaccinated with the HPV vaccine, have a discussion with your health care provider. Examine the risks and benefits of the vaccine, and the risks and benefits of not getting the vaccine. If you choose against the vaccine, then it is important to make sure that PAP smears are started within three years of becoming sexually active and continue every one to two years.

Adult Vaccines
Vaccinations are continued throughout the lifespan. Once again, which vaccines you choose or choose not to receive should be discussed with your health care provider. While most vaccines have been proven to be safe, there are times when your health care provider may recommend that you forgo them. The cases in which your health care provider may recommend delaying or forgoing the vaccines are; if you are taking

medications that weaken your immune system, have certain medical conditions and/or are pregnant. Below are some of the more common vaccines that adults may be encouraged to get during their lifetime.

Flu Vaccines

The seasonal flu vaccine generally changes every year based on the strain of flu that is predominate in any given flu season. Occasionally, as with the H1N1 flu, you will see more than one strain circulating. There are times when these differing strains can be combined into one seasonal vaccine, but there are other times when that is not possible, and your health care provider may recommend more than one vaccine. While flu vaccines are good at decreasing the number of flu cases, they are not 100 percent guaranteed. It is possible to still get the flu after you have been vaccinated. Occasionally, you will have been exposed to the virus before the vaccine has had time to develop antibodies in your system. Other times, you may get the flu, but the symptoms will be less severe than had you not been vaccinated. Certainly if you are over 65 years old and/or have chronic medical problems you should make sure that you get vaccinated every flu season.

Pneumonia Vaccine

The pneumonia vaccine is generally recommended for patients 65 years of age and older and/or those with chronic lung problems, respiratory diseases, cardiac issues as well as smokers and patients with a history of spleen removal. This vaccine is generally given every 5 years. While there are over 80 known types of pneumococcus bacterium, the current vaccine protects against the 23 most common strains. The vaccine also does not protect against the viral strains of pneumonia. While this vaccine does not insure that a recipient won't get some form of pneumonia, it does lessen the chance and usually the severity of the disease. If you or a loved one lives in a retirement, assisted living or nursing facility, it is highly recommended that you have this vaccine. Areas where people live in close proximity to each other increase the spread of bacteria such as pneumonia.

Tetanus/Diphtheria Vaccine
The tetanus vaccine is recommended for almost everyone. This
vaccine is given generally every ten years to prevent tetanus from
skin wounds. If you have a particularly dirty wound, your health
care provider may recommend a vaccine after 5 years. If you cannot
remember when your last tetanus vaccine was, it won't hurt you to get
another. In the case of tetanus it is better to be safe than sorry.

Recently they have started adding a pertussis booster to some of the
tetanus vaccines. Pertussis is more commonly known as whooping
cough and is caused by the Bordetella bacteria. In recent years, there
has been an increase in the number of adult cases of whooping cough,
and disease specialists saw a need to have adults receive this booster
at some point between the ages of 11-64 years of age. People with the
highest risk of contracting pertussis are those with exposure to young
children. If you receive the tetanus vaccine with the pertussis booster,
make sure to make a note of it in your vaccination log so that you can
inform future health care providers that you have already received the
booster and when.

Shingles Vaccine
Shingles is a very painful condition caused by the same virus that
causes Chickenpox. You have to have had Chickenpox to develop
Shingles. Shingles will generally develop along the nerves in the
upper torso, head and face and can occasionally cause permanent
damage and pain. To lessen your chance of Shingles it is recommended
that you get the Shingles vaccine after the age of 60.

You and your health care provider can make decisions together
regarding your vaccination schedule. Although vaccines have been
deemed relatively safe, side effects may occur. They are generally mild
and localized at the site of injection. Localized reactions generally
involve itching, redness, swelling, warmth, soreness and stiffness. It is
also possible to have mild systemic reactions such as low grade fever,
achiness and mild flu-like symptoms. Usually there is no reason to be
alarmed or contact your health care provider for mild reactions. For
more severe reactions, such as redness and swelling that continues

to worsen, high fevers, difficulty breathing, mental and neurological symptoms, you should contact your health care provider or seek emergency treatment.

Generally, health maintenance and disease prevention is an ongoing process. Below are some other measures that you can take to reduce your chances of disease contraction and increase your health maintenance.

Oral Health

Regular visits to the dentist are also an integral part of health maintenance and disease prevention. Good oral health practices can prevent decay and/or infection and can lead to early onset disease detection. Visiting your dentist every 6 to 12 months for a thorough cleaning and exam can help insure not only good dental health, but also overall health maintenance. Gum disease and dental decay that goes unchecked, can result in decreased nutritional intake and increased risks of localized or systemic infections.

In addition to dental visits, a regular routine of brushing, flossing and dietary maintenance can insure greater dental health and overall health maintenance. There are a number of things that can lead to dental issues such as consuming items containing high sugar content, highly acidic foods and drinks, tobacco products, certain teeth whitening products, coffee, teas and sodas. Use your dentist as a good resource for the best dental products and the safest whitening and cosmetic products.

Antibacterial Products

There are many of these products on the market. For the most part, they are very beneficial at slowing or stopping the spread of germs. As an emergency room nurse, I have found the antibacterial hand cleaners to be not only a figurative, but a literal life saver. As a health care provider, I have found that they increase compliance with hand washing between patients and procedures and save time during the course of a shift. While these products are beneficial, there are times when a thorough hand washing with soap and water is still required. If your hands are visibly soiled or have contacted any bodily fluids, soap and water is still the preferred method. Certainly, if you are working with meat products when cooking, hand washing before and after is a must.

While antibacterial products are a wonderful addition to our health maintenance practices, as with anything else, too much of a good thing can be a bad thing. Some studies have shown that people who have become obsessed with bacterial elimination, have in turn destroyed an important part of their immune protection. There are certain bacteria that live not only on our skin, but also in our internal systems. These bacteria are referred to as normal flora. While generally this normal flora is beneficial to our immune process, there are times when they can wreak havoc. When people become overly obsessed with removing all the bacteria in their environment, they eliminate the body's ability to fight infections and diseases. So, when disinfecting yourself and your environment, keep balance in mind. If you eliminate all the bacteria in your environment, your immune system will be less likely to build resistance and maintain a healthy and normal bacterial balance.

Environmental Toxins
While it is almost humanly impossible to avoid exposure to the multitudes of environmental toxins, it is possible to reduce your exposure through awareness and diligence. Below is a list of some of the common toxins in our environment and ways to reduce your exposure.

Food products
Whether it is fruits, vegetables, meat, dairy products, packaged or processed foods, all contain at least trace levels of some environmental toxins. To decrease exposure, try to buy organic when possible and affordable. Keep in mind that even organically grown and raised foods still have trace toxins due to air pollution and ground water contamination. While it is virtually impossible to find food without

some contamination, your exposure will be greatly decreased going the organic route. When you are purchasing processed and packaged foods pay attention to ingredients and additives to further decrease your exposure. If you can't pronounce the ingredients, chances are you don't want to eat it.

Water

Most communities have water treatment plants that keep our water supply relatively safe, but even with treatment there are trace amounts of chemicals and toxins that slip through to your water faucet. Recently, there have been reports of traces of medications in the public water supply that come from health care facilities, manufacturers and the public flushing old and unused medications into the sewage systems. To avoid the contaminants in the public water supply, people turn to buying bottled water in plastic bottles. The plastic bottles often come with their own set of toxins. What are you to do if you want a clean drink of water? As stated earlier, it is probably impossible to avoid all exposure, but using a water filter, drinking out of safe materials and being personally responsible to what you contribute to the public water supply will help to decrease your personal exposure.

Dishes and Containers

Another area of exposure to contaminants is the dishes, cookware and storage containers we use in the kitchen. To avoid higher exposures to these contaminants, know what you are using and when and how to use it. Some dishes and china have lead components that can seep into the foods. The dishes with the highest levels of lead are generally older and become discolored when exposed to the heat of modern dishwashers and microwaves. Limit your use of these types of dishes and avoid reheating food in them in microwaves if you suspect the dishes contain lead components. Also avoid reheating foods in the microwave in the plastic storage containers. The heat of microwaves increases the release of the chemicals contained within the plastics. There have also been concerns about the chemicals used in non-stick cooking surfaces, so decrease your exposure by using cast iron or stainless steel vessels when possible.

Lawn and Garden Chemicals
This is another area where there is concern for toxic exposures. If using organic compounds and materials is not an option, then take appropriate precautions when handling these substances. Wear gloves, masks and protective clothing when working with lawn and garden chemicals, store them appropriately, clean up spills and dispose of the chemicals properly.

Elective and Non-elective Procedures
The final area of health maintenance discussed in this chapter surrounds the decisions of whether or not to participate in elective and non-elective procedures and surgeries. The difference between elective procedures and non-elective procedures is that elective procedures may enhance your life in some way, but is not necessary in order to maintain or save your life. Non-elective procedures are required to maintain life or quality of life. While most elective procedures have a relatively high degree of safety, all of them carry a certain amount of risk even when performed properly. This is why you are asked to sign an informed consent before even the most benign procedures. The informed consent will generally state that you were made aware of the inherent risks of a procedure. Regardless the procedure, it is important to understand the risks presented, and if they are not presented to you, make sure you ask the provider what the risks are.

Elective procedures can be something as simple as hair removal or as complex as plastic surgery requiring general anesthetic and everything in between. When choosing an elective procedure, think carefully about what the benefits are and how important it is to the quality of your life. Even the simplest cosmetic procedures can come with serious inherent risks including infection and disfiguration. Other risks involved in elective procedures include adverse reactions to anesthesia, blood clots and cardiac events. Once you have decided to proceed, check the qualifications of the person providing the services. For example, some cosmetic procedures are provided by people who are not medical providers. These people should be certified or licensed by a cosmetology board or another governing board that helps to insure quality and safety. Always check qualifications and experience before proceeding with any elective procedure.

When facing a non-elective surgery, it is advisable to get a second opinion when possible. Except in extreme emergency or life saving situations, there is generally time to get a second opinion to make sure that it is the surgery you need and that you have the person you want performing it. An example to illustrate this point involves a nurse friend of mine, who had several ruptured discs in her neck. She worked in the surgery department and knew an older surgeon whom she had worked with for several years and trusted implicitly. She consulted with him and he stated that in order to fix all the levels involved it would require two procedures at least six months apart. The problem was, the first procedure would only fix half the problem and the pain that she was experiencing would continue for another six months while waiting for the second procedure. During the same time, I was working on a floor that had patients with the same problem who were having surgery by a younger doctor who used a newer procedure. The results were remarkable and the patients experienced very little post-operative pain. I suggested she consult with this younger doctor to see if he could fix all the levels in one procedure. She was hesitant to obtain the second opinion, feeling a sense of loyalty to the first doctor. She finally relinquished, got the second opinion and was able to get the problem fixed with one surgery with excellent results. In this case, the patient saved herself and her insurance company the costs of having a second operation. More importantly, she lowered her risks by having only one procedure. She was also able to return to work sooner saving lost wages.

When faced with a non-elective surgery, it is important to always follow the example of getting a second opinion. Having worked in the health care field for many years, I have seen many surgeons go straight to the surgery option versus other available treatments and options. The main reason is that surgery is their business and they don't make anything if someone chooses a non-surgical method. As stated before, most health care providers do the right thing most of the time, but no one cares more about your health than you do, and a good surgeon will concur that you should obtain a second opinion.

Once you have determined that surgery is the option, then make sure that your surgeon is the right one for the job. Once again, do your research. Talk to your friends, other health care providers and get online to check the surgeon's performance record. Also, make sure that the surgeon has privileges at the hospital of your choice. There are hospitals that perform better in some areas than in others. If you are facing an outpatient procedure this aspect may not be as important, but should always be a consideration. Many outpatient surgeries are now being done at outpatient surgery centers. These centers are generally very good at doing what they do, but make sure to ask how they are equipped to deal with the unexpected. While most outpatient surgeries done in these independent, free standing centers have a relatively high level of safety, emergencies do crop up and they should be prepared to handle the immediate emergency and have a policy in place to transfer a patient out if needed. Always ask where patients are transferred in case of emergency, and make sure that fits into your health care plans.

Of course, the best laid plans can get blown up by insurance issues. While insurance may not even be a concern with some elective procedures and most cosmetic procedures, it will make a difference with non-elective procedures. Check your plan and the providers covered before starting your research. It makes no sense to research a health care provider for non-elective procedures who does not work with your insurance coverage.

Chapter 7

Disease Management

Sometimes we can do all the right things in terms of health maintenance and still succumb to some form of disease process. Depending
on the disease or condition, the management of disease processes can
become daunting. Throughout the chapter, we will cover some of the
most common disease processes and keys to disease management. Of
course, this chapter will be a rather general overview considering the
massive number of diseases, conditions and therapies.

As discussed in the Health Maintenance section, many disease
processes are a result of lifestyle choices, genetic predispositions and/
or environmental exposures. The diseases resulting from lifestyle
choices can, of course, be reversed or managed through the changing
of lifestyle. Those stemming from genetic predispositions can also be
managed somewhat in the fact that knowledge is power, and knowing
your genetic tendencies allows you to be more aware and proactive.
Diseases resulting from environmental exposures are sometimes more
tenuous in that you don't always know what you are being exposed to.

To start, we will discuss some of the keys to managing disease
processes through prescription medications and the things you should
do to insure the highest degree of safety and effectiveness.

Is a prescription right for you?
Once your health care provider has diagnosed a disease process, the
first step is generally a prescription to treat or cure. A prescription

may be the easiest way of treating the problem, but is it the best? Don't be afraid to ask this question. All medications come with side effects and drawbacks. These side effects may lead to additional prescriptions down the road. Ask your health care provider if there are alternative treatments. Some alternatives could include lifestyle changes, natural methods, or perhaps some sort of disease counseling.

Know your medications

The most important thing to do once your health care provider prescribes a medication, is to know what the medication is and what it is for. Ask the health care provider to give you both the trade name and the generic name and ask for at least a simplified explanation of how the medication works. It is also important to know the dosage of the medication and how many times a day you should take it. Pay attention to the prescription and know the difference between milligrams and micrograms. The abbreviations are similar, milligrams (mg) and micrograms (mcg). While the abbreviations are similar, there is a huge difference in the dosage. Learn about your medication either from your health care provider or pharmacist or both. Know the best time of day to take it, what foods or drinks may interact with the medication, and, most importantly, know what the side effects are. Learn how to determine if the medication is performing as it should. Is the medication making you better or worse?

Keep your health care provider informed

Once diagnosed with a disease process, make sure that you keep your health care provider well informed of changes in how you feel, changes in your lifestyle and changes in your nutritional and over-the-counter supplements. It is common for people to think that if they are taking any sort of health food, nutritional and/or vitamin supplement, they do not need to inform their health care provider. The fact is that many of these products are not regulated in this country and many, even if natural, can cause adverse reactions with many medications and conditions. We have already discussed how garlic can increase your bleeding times, so if you are taking blood thinning medications and eating a lot of foods high in garlic, you may be increasing your risks of bleeding disorders. All of your care providers should be aware of anything that you are taking or doing that can have a positive or negative impact on your disease management.

Start your list
Make the list we talked about earlier. List all of your medications by both names, the dosages, how many times per day you take them and when you started taking each one. Keep this list up to date and with you at all times. Unfortunately, we don't always know when we may make an unexpected trip to an urgent care or emergency room. If you don't know the medication or the dosage or when you started taking the medication, your treatment plan may be adversely affected. The advantage of having a written list is that nothing is left to chance. When faced with an emergency, you may have trouble remembering and/or be unable to speak for yourself, so having your medications in writing will assist your health care providers. Many medications sound alike so it is helpful for the medical provider to have the proper spelling of your medications.

What can happen without this list? Let's say that you go to the emergency room and you don't have a list of medications. The medical staff is going to ask you for your medications. You answer the best you can, but you cannot remember the dose of one medication. You tell them that you think it is 50 mg. In actuality, the dose is 25 mg twice a day. The medical provider will list the medication as 50 mg twice a day. You then get admitted to the hospital and the entry follows you. You are now going to receive double the dose needed. Worse yet, the doctor discharges you home on that dose, gives you a new prescription for the wrong dose, and nobody notices. In the case of a medication for high blood pressure, or any medication for that matter, it could have rather devastating results. Using the blood pressure medication as an example, you are now taking a double dose and can't figure out why you are so tired or keep passing out after feeling dizzy. You go back to your doctor or hospital and incur additional testing, treatment and medical costs, all of which could be avoided by keeping an accurate list with you at all times.

Know the history of your medication

Is the medication that your health care provider prescribed a drug
that has been on the market for a while or is it a new one? Both have
advantages and disadvantages. A medication that has been on the
market for several years is usually well proven and cheaper. Newer
medications may be improved versions, but may not have been tested
as extensively in the general population and will be more expensive
because of patent issues. Once a medication's patent expires, the price
drops dramatically. Many pharmaceutical companies and health care
providers will heavily promote newer medications without telling you
that the mechanism of action is basically the same. In some cases,
when a drug's patent runs out, the manufacturer will change the
chemical structure just slightly to generate a new patent, slap a new
name on it and be able to once again charge a premium price for basically the same medication. In the end, it will be your wallet that will
take a big hit. On other occasions, new medications are produced that
may treat a disease better with fewer side effects. Ask your medical
provider, and then ask your pharmacist. A good pharmacist can be
your best source of information.

Be consistent and compliant

Once you and your health care provider have decided on a medication,
make sure that you take it as prescribed as often as possible. There
are reasons that pharmaceutical companies and health care providers
prescribe medications on the schedules they do. Some medications
work most effectively when taken every few hours, while others can be
taken once a day. Other medications take a while to build up a therapeutic level in your blood stream and should not be stopped abruptly.
Missing a single dose is generally not a problem and you can get back
on schedule with the next dose, but before stopping a medication,
always check with your health care provider. Unless it is a case of a
significant allergic reaction, your medical provider may make recommendations for weaning from a medication.

Let's look at some of the more common medications and the compliance issues that many patients face.

Antibiotics

Antibiotics are prescribed for any number of bacterial infections. Health care providers will prescribe antibiotics based on the bacteria that are the common cause for specific infections. Sometimes a health care provider will run tests to determine the exact bacteria causing the infection. In the meantime, he will prescribe the most common antibiotic for that infection, and when he gets the tests results back, may change the antibiotic to one that the bacteria is most susceptible to. When possible, it is best to wait for the results to come back so the patient is started on the most appropriate medication. When a patient is too sick to wait, it is better to start on something that will at least provide some general coverage until more information is garnered. Once the information is collected, the patient may be asked to change antibiotics. Patients should properly dispose of any remaining antibiotics before starting the more specific one. Unfortunately, when this scenario happens, many people will keep the first antibiotic in the medicine cabinet for possible future use. There are a couple problems with this plan. First, a patient may get another type of infection and start taking the antibiotic on hand to avoid an additional doctor's visit. Since all antibiotics are not created equally, this is almost always a bad idea. An antibiotic that is not specific to the infection will not help and will probably make matters worse. Second, antibiotics, as most medications, have assigned expiration dates. Overtime a medication's potency will either decrease or increase resulting in inappropriate dosage concentrations.

Another compliance issue with antibiotics is patients will quit taking them when they start to feel better. What results is the antibiotic has only had the opportunity to kill the weakest of the bacteria, and the stronger or more stubborn bacteria remain in the body just to rear their ugly heads at a later date. When this happens, these bacteria will be more resistant to future treatment. When you are taking antibiotics, make sure to take them as scheduled and until they are completely gone to reduce the risk of reoccurrence and resistance.

Refrain from taking antibiotics prescribed for someone else even if for the same symptoms. As stated earlier, not all bacteria are created equal and taking a partial prescription will lead to ineffective treatment, resistance and increased risk of worsening infection.

A final note on antibiotic therapy, antibiotics are used for the treatment of bacterial infections. Colds and flus are caused by viruses, yet many patients will go to their health care providers and demand an antibiotic. Unfortunately, many health care providers will prescribe the antibiotics to keep their patients happy. Not only is this dangerous for the patient, because the antibiotics will destroy the patient's normal flora, but it is also dangerous for the general patient population, because the antibiotics will become less effective overall. Make sure that you have a thorough discussion with your health care provider before starting antibiotic therapy.

High blood pressure (hypertension) medications

This is another group of medications that patients have demonstrated compliance issues with. When patients are diagnosed with high blood pressure and treated with prescription medications, many patients will, after a few normal readings, stop taking the medications thinking that their disease no longer exists. This can lead to some dire consequences with increased risks of stroke and cardiovascular events. There are times that with appropriate lifestyle changes patients can get their blood pressure under control, but stopping the medication should only be done under medical supervision.

Yet another compliance issue revolves around patients deciding to increase or double up on their blood pressure medications if they feel that their blood pressure is high. This too can lead to disastrous results. Patients should always check with their health care provider before increasing their dosages to avoid undiagnosed problems or overdose situations.

Depression and anxiety medications

While there are some medications that can control acute and/or severe attacks of anxiety with a one time dose, most of the medications prescribed for chronic anxiety and depression have to be taken for a period of time before they truly become therapeutic. Once again, many patients will start to feel better and stop taking the medications or only take them when they are feeling depressed or anxious. These medications are not effective when taken this way and can lead to more serious bouts of depression and anxiety, and in the worse case scenarios can lead to suicidal thoughts and actions. If a patient feels that she no longer needs these medications then she should contact her medical provider and get a schedule for slowly weaning off these medications.

Steroids

Steroids are a class of medications used to treat a number of conditions including respiratory infections, asthma, allergic reactions, pain and inflammation. These medications can have major consequences for many other organ systems including insulin levels, blood pressure, etc. Many times these medications are started at high doses and then gradually lowered. It is once again advisable to follow the directions on taking, weaning and stopping these medications to avoid adverse effects.

Insulin

Problems may also occur for those taking insulin, especially when people take both the short acting and long acting insulin. The problem is that the insulin vials are generally very small and similar in appearance. Many patients will grab the wrong vial, and they will end up taking the wrong dose of the wrong medication. To avoid this problem, patients should make distinct markings on the vials or keep a magnifying glass present to make sure that they are grabbing the right vial. Diligence with insulin is very important to avoid a trip to the emergency room.

Blood Thinners

Blood thinning medications are a group of medications that can cause very serious problems if you do not exercise compliance. There are many common foods and over-the-counter medications that increase the efficiency of blood thinning medications which can cause life threatening bleeding conditions. When taking these medications, it is important to comply with frequent follow ups with your health care provider to check bleeding times to ensure the blood thinners are within their therapeutic levels.

Over-the-Counter Medications

Many people believe that if you can buy something over-the-counter then it must be safe. While most over-the-counter medications have a high degree of safety, there are always potential problems. It is imperative that if you take any prescription medications, you check with your pharmacist about any possible interactions with over-the-counter medications. One problem that is often seen is people take narcotic pain medications and then take over-the-counter pain medications. Many of these medications contain the same active ingredients. The pharmaceutical companies are now starting to change the formulas of the prescription medications to avoid some of the overdose potentials, but continue to check with your pharmacist and/or health care provider. Another problem with over-the-counter medications is encountered by patients who suffer from high blood pressure and/or heart disease. Many of the cold, flu and allergy medications sold over-the-counter can increase blood pressure and heart rate.

While there are many beneficial over-the-counter medications, before taking any of them follow a few common sense precautions. First, read the label carefully to familiarize yourself with the ingredients and the label warnings. Secondly, ask your health care provider about what over-the-counter medications may interact with your prescription medications. Thirdly, consult your local pharmacist for recommendations based on your prescriptions and medical history. And finally, treat over-the-counter medications as you would prescription medications and supplements, and keep a list of the ones that you take on a regular basis.

Regardless of the medication, compliance and consistency is the key to achieving the greatest therapeutic effects. There are several ways to achieve these goals. First, purchase a container that is divided into the seven days of the week and different day parts. At the beginning of the week, you load up your medications and can keep track of when you took your last medication and when your next medication is due. Many of these containers are divided into daily sleeves so that you can take just the one sleeve with you for that day. Secondly, you can purchase medication watches that have alarms that can be set to go off several times a day to remind you to take the medications, or you can set the alarm on your cell phone to provide a reminder. And finally, if all else fails, keep a little notebook with you to mark down the times and medications as you take them.

Know the difference between allergic reactions and adverse reactions. It is important to distinguish the difference between these two reactions. Allergic reactions can simply be annoying with itching, hives and redness or life threatening with respiratory system involvement and shock. Regardless of the severity of the allergic reaction, you should put this on your medication list as an official allergy to avoid future complications. Adverse reactions are basically side effects of the medications. If you have a truly undesired side effect of a medication, then you would want to list this as an allergy as well. Keep in mind that many medications have side effects that we may not necessarily prefer, but the advantages of the medications outweigh the adverse reactions. For example, many of the chemotherapy agents used in cancer treatments have many adverse effects, but their benefits generally outweigh these effects.

Make sure everybody is on the same page
This is probably the most important piece of advice. When your health care provider writes a prescription for you, make sure to question her about the name, the proper enunciation, the reasons for taking it, the side effects, cross allergies, dosages and frequencies. This may sound redundant, but remember that your health care provider is seeing a number of patients in the course of a day and you want to make sure her mind is on you. Asking these questions will provide a

cue to the health care provider to make sure that she is on the same page that you are. Once you are sure that you and your health care provider are on the same page make sure that your pharmacy is right there with you. Always check for your name, the medication name and dosage. Pharmacies can be very busy places and there are times when the wrong person walks out with the wrong medication. The other problem that may crop up is the pharmacist may not be able to read the health care provider's hand writing. Many medication names look alike when scribbled. Ask the pharmacist the same questions mentioned above to double check. The good news here is that many health care providers are going to electronic prescriptions which are easier for everyone to read. While technology is cutting down on some of the handwriting mistakes, there are of course, mistakes that can be electronically generated. When generating an electronic prescription health care providers usually pick from a list of medications so it is possible for them to click the wrong medication. Be your own best advocate and double check everything before popping that pill into your mouth.

Let's now take a look at ways you can advocate for yourself or a family member if faced with one of the more common diagnoses we see in the health care field today.

Alzheimer's Disease

Alzheimer's disease is a complicated disease to manage both as a patient and/or caregiver. There are different degrees of severity and almost as many different presentations as there are individuals who are affected. This disease is still, in many ways, a mystery to the medical profession in terms of prevention and prediction of who will succumb. The disease has been linked to certain lifestyle choices, environmental exposures and genetics. The fact is that no one can predict with any degree of certainty who will get it, when they will get it or why they will get it. With Alzheimer's there is no cure, but there are certain things patients can do to prolong functionality.

Alzheimer's is a disease that often creeps up on people. It is a gradual and progressive disease that steals your memory, health and independence. Diagnosing Alzheimer's is not easy; at this time the only way to definitively diagnose the disease is by examining the brain after death. Most health care professionals will diagnose the disease after other causes of symptoms have been eliminated. Many things can mimic some of the signs of Alzheimer's including heart disease, vascular problems, neurological problems, infectious processes, electrolyte imbalances, hormonal imbalances, psychiatric processes, sleep disturbances and of course lifestyle. Memory deficits are one of the first things that come to mind when people think of Alzheimer's. So if you forgot where you put your keys this morning should you be concerned? Probably not, this type of memory issue is generally related to being hurried, having too many things on your mind or just simply a momentary loss of concentration. If these incidents increase in frequency and intensity, and happen several times throughout the day, every day, then you will want to see your health care provider for a further evaluation.

While it is difficult to accurately predict the speed in which Alzheimer's will progress, there has been some promising work in that area. The tests that are showing promise are based on baseline memory status measured over time and rate of decline. Because the rate of progression is different for each individual, it is important to find a health care professional who can monitor the patient on a regular basis. Proper, continuous monitoring can help both the individual and family plan accordingly in relationship to future health care needs, life care needs and financial considerations.

There is no way to definitely predict if you are at risk for Alzheimer's and no significant preventive measures. As with many disease processes discussed in this chapter it comes down to lifestyle changes and/or genetics. There has been some evidence to show that regular mental exercises such as word puzzles and memory games can prolong mental function. There have also been several medications developed that help preserve and prolong the memory and thought processes.

Once an individual has received a diagnosis of Alzheimer's, it can be devastating not only to the patient, but to family and friends. Early in the diagnostic process is the time to take stock of your life. If you have not done your medical legal documents, do them. Talk with not only your health care providers, but have open and honest conversations with family and friends about your expectations and desires related to future care and financial issues. Discuss issues such as long term care options, medical treatment and end of life planning. Alzheimer's is a disease that in and of itself will not result in death. Death is usually a result of related issues caused by wandering, falling, home accidents and nutritional imbalances related to forgetting to eat or forgetting that you have already eaten. This disease can go on for years and even decades providing innumerable challenges to the patient, family, care-givers and health care providers.

Dealing with the challenges of Alzheimer's is a difficult process. Often the patient has moments of extreme clarity followed by moments of extreme confusion and personality changes. One key to dealing with Alzheimer's is to keep the patient safe. There have been many advancements to help keep the Alzheimer's patient safe. Technological advancements in GPS monitoring, home alarm and monitoring services and computer camera technology can provide methods to monitor the patient without smothering. There are several other things that you can do to manage this disease process:

1. The best place to start is the Alzheimer Foundation's web site at **www.alzfdn.org.** This web site will provide invaluable resources for planning and caring for the Alzheimer's patient. It also provides hints on where to find care-giving help and support.

2. Join a support group. Joining a support group can help you feel less alone. Members of the group will often share their successes and fail-ures, helping you avoid learning from trial and error.

3. Start focusing on safety. Monitor driving abilities, and when they start to decline take action such as prohibiting access to keys, licenses and cars. Keep in mind that the Alzheimer's patient will have

moments of amazing clarity and problem solving abilities. An example is a patient we saw in the ER after she became disoriented and lost. She was found wandering in the parking lot looking for her car and was becoming increasingly agitated. Concerned citizens called for an emergency squad who brought her to the ER. Once her daughter showed up, she told of how she took her mother's keys and license from her to prevent her from driving. The patient, in one of those moments of clarity, called the car dealership and told them that she had lost her keys and needed a new set delivered. The dealership, not knowing any better, brought her the keys and that was all it took for her to get behind the wheel again. Needless to say, the daughter ended up confiscating the car. Keep in mind that losing the ability to drive is a huge hit to a patient's feeling of independence and will be a difficult challenge to confront. Be patient yet adamant, once that day comes not only for the patient's safety, but also the public's safety.

4. Inform neighbors, family and friends of the situation so they can notify the appropriate person if the patient starts to wander.

5. Look into patient and home monitoring options.

6. Ensure that the patient's financial resources are being closely monitored to prevent the patient from being scammed and removing large sums of money from accounts without remembering.

7. Decide whether the patient is able to be cared for at home or needs to be placed in an extended care facility, day care facility or provided with home health assistance. There is no right answer for this dilemma. Deciding the level of care will depend on the patient's abilities and resources of caregivers. While many patients think staying in their own home is the best option, and the caregivers will think they are able to provide the level of care required, it may not always be the best choice. Daycare facilities and extended care facilities can sometimes provide more continuous stimulation and closer and safer monitoring of the patient than would be physically possible for the patient to receive in a private home setting. The other concern, is whether the caregiver is able to provide the required level of care without suffering

himself or hurting the patient? In severe cases, safety is always a
concern. Many families are afraid to go to sleep, because they have
been awakened by fires or floods in the home.

When looking at safety issues, start with a floor to ceiling assessment
of the home. Think of it as childproofing for a very tall child. It may
be appropriate at times to regulate the power supply of appliances
such as stoves and microwaves. An Alzheimer's patient will forget that
appliances are on or how to use them properly and safely.

8. Most importantly, if you become a caregiver for the Alzheimer's
patient, remember not to take it personally. Because this disease robs
people of their minds and personalities, these patients will often not
remember the ones closest to them, and may demonstrate a personality far different from their baseline.

Anxiety

Anxiety is becoming an alarmingly prevalent diagnosis. The economy,
global issues, personal relationships, work stress, and many other
things are at the root of many patients' anxiety. If you have ever
suffered an anxiety or panic attack, you know how unnerving it can
be. Since anxiety can mimic many other conditions such as asthma,
stroke and heart disease, it is important to have these symptoms
evaluated and to not just ignore them.

The symptoms of anxiety and panic can be quite frightening and
manifest themselves in a very real physical presentation. Some of the
symptoms include chest pain, palpitations, dizziness, lightheadedness,
difficulty breathing from chest or throat tightening, sweating, nausea,
hyperventilation, dry mouth, increased blood pressure, distorted
perceptions, overwhelming sense of doom, preoccupation with symptoms and fear of dying. Depending on the degree of anxiety these
symptoms can range from mild to severe.

The treatment of anxiety should be individualized and multifaceted. The first step in the treatment process should be an evaluation
of the source of anxiety. Is the anxiety being caused by situational

circumstances such as mentioned above, chemical or hormonal imbalances and/or dietary origins? Unfortunately, many times anxiety is misdiagnosed, treated only by medications and/or ignored or downplayed by health care providers. If you find yourself suffering from an anxiety/panic disorder, you must be proactive in advocating for yourself and making sure you are getting the appropriate treatment for the type and level of anxiety that you are experiencing. Without appropriate diagnosis and treatment, anxiety can devastate your life and relationships.

In severe acute cases of anxiety often caused by extreme life situations, a short term course of sedative-type medications may be all that is needed. In more chronic cases of anxiety, an anti-anxiety medication may be prescribed. In this case, it is important to continue to try to get to the root cause of the anxiety, which may involve investigating counseling, chemical and hormonal testing, tracking your dietary intake, reviewing other medications, and evaluating your alcohol or drug use. Once a cause is identified, then you are at a point where you can discuss treatment options with your health care provider. Some alternatives to medication regimes may include continued counseling, biofeedback, exercise, weight loss, diet control, meditation and avoidance of stimulants.

Arthritis
Arthritis is one of those pesky disease processes that creep up on just about everyone at some point in life. There are of course ways to minimize the damage that this joint disease can cause. As with just about everything, diet and exercise can help stave it off for a while. In the case of arthritis, all exercise is not created equal. There are several activities that can wear the joints out faster than others. Generally, a sound weight bearing exercise such as walking combined with a strength and flexibility workout work best at keeping the joints and surrounding tissues in a healthy state. Jogging, running and high impact activities tend to wear the joints out a little faster. Recreational activities such as racquet sports and court sports can also take their toll on joints. The better your underlying condition when participating in these activities, the more you will be able to prolong your overall joint health.

When the pain and stiffness start, there are several supplemental regimes that you can begin to provide pain relief, reduce some of the associated stiffness and prolong remaining joint health. The one supplement that has become popular over the past decade is the glucosamine and chondroitin combination that helps to maintain the cushioning in the joints. The other supplements that help with healthy joints are vitamin D and calcium. And of course, one of my favorites is the apple cider vinegar with the Mother (the sediment). Drink one teaspoon in eight ounces of water three times a day.

The next step if the above measures don't work is to start taking one of the over-the-counter non-steroidal anti-inflammatory medications, analgesics and/or medicated analgesic pain patches. While all of these things are sold over-the-counter, care should still be taken in the decision making process and usage. In the case of the non-steroidal anti-inflammatory medications (NSAIDS), many of them can cause stomach ulcers, bleeding disorders, increased risk of cardiovascular incidents and, with prolonged therapy, an increase in blood pressure. Take them only as recommended and on an occasional basis. Other analgesics such as aspirin and acetaminophen are in many other over-the-counter medications such as cold and flu medications. Make sure to always check the labels on all of your over-the-counter medications to make sure you are not exceeding the recommended dosages. The same warnings apply to the analgesic patches. It is possible to absorb too much of the medication contained in the patches if you leave them on too long or use too many of them. Make sure that when you remove the patches you wipe off the medications with soap and water and follow application and usage instructions.

When everything else has failed and your arthritis is starting to impact your daily quality of life, it may be time to visit a health care provider such as your family doctor and/or and orthopedic surgeon. There are several prescription anti-inflammatory medications and, in the worst case scenario, there are narcotic pain medications to help with pain relief. The prescription medications come with many of the same side effects, and with long term use of narcotics, an increase in the risk for addiction issues. Your doctor may also prescribe physical therapy to strengthen surrounding muscles to prolong your remaining joint health. There are also several things that your doctor can inject right into the joint to decrease swelling and provide pain relief. If these tactics don't work and you find yourself unable to do the things that you enjoy doing, surgery may be the next step. Advocating for yourself in this scenario requires asking several questions:

1. Have we tried all other available alternatives?

2. What are the risks and benefits of the surgical procedure? While there are thousands of joint surgeries done safely and without complications every day in this country, all surgeries come with risks. When these risks rear their ugly heads, it is possible to end up in worse shape than when you started. Make sure that you are well informed before undertaking this step.

3. Are there any new techniques or approaches available? Things change fast in health care. There are new surgical techniques developed every day such as laser techniques, microsurgeries and robotic procedures. Many of the newer techniques come with the benefits of quicker recover times, better pain control, decreased risk of infection and less scarring. Ask your surgeon if she uses any of the newer technologies. Keep in mind, surgeons who are resistant to change may not provide some of the newer techniques. Do your research on what is available and who in your area does it. When time permits, always try to get a second opinion.

4. Do you need a total or partial joint replacement? Sometimes it is possible to replace just part of a joint maintaining as much of the original joint as possible.

5. How long will the procedure or joint last?

6. What are the surgeon's post-operative infection rates?

7. What are the hospital/surgery center's post-operative infection rates? As with anything in life, there are some people and some places

that just get the job done better than others. Make sure that you have the best when possible. There are many websites available to check these rates in your area. You can also check with friends and family members who have had a good experience. If you have friends or family members who work in the health care field, ask them who they would go to or not go to, they usually have the inside scoop.

8. What are the surgeon's post-operative complication rates?

9. How well equipped is the facility to handle unexpected emergencies?

10. What is the estimated recovery time?

11. What will the post-operative limitations be?

12. What kind of post-operative follow-up is provided and for how long?

13. What will your insurance cover for the different options?

Once you have the answers to the above questions, you should be able to make a well informed decision. Just keep in mind that all surgeries come with risks. Make sure that your surgeon is educated and trained in the most recent and sound procedures. And finally, make sure you have thoroughly investigated all of your choices.

Asthma
Asthma is a disease process that affects many people in many different ways. Asthma can be both an acute and chronic disease process. Regardless of whether or not the asthma is a result of an acute or chronic process, it can be a very frightening experience causing chest tightness, shortness of breath and in severe cases a complete inability to breathe.

Acute asthma can result from a number of things including bron-chitis, upper respiratory infections, environmental factors, and food exposures. Even though acute asthma is a temporary condition, it can still be quite serious and requires early medical intervention to avoid life threatening events. If asthma is caused by environmental factors, it is of course best to avoid those things that trigger it. Because this is not always possible, it is imperative to talk with your health care provider about emergency medications to carry with you in case of an exposure. Keep these medications current by regularly checking the expirations dates. In severe cases of environmentally induced asthma attacks, it is a good idea to wear a medic alert bracelet or chain to aid in treatment in emergency situations. If you contract a particularly bad upper respiratory infection, bronchitis or have an acute asthma attack for any reason, a visit to your health care provider is warranted to prevent a life threatening situation. Once the infection clears up or the exposure is diminished, the asthma will likely clear up as well.

Chronic asthma is often present from childhood on, but can develop at any time throughout the lifespan. The best way to deal with chronic asthma is to work closely with your health care provider to keep it under control and to keep severe attacks to a minimum. If you suffer from chronic asthma, you probably can tell when a severe attack is imminent. It is important when you feel an attack coming on to seek medical attention before it gets too out of control. There has been some recent research into the effect that diet has on asthma and some correlation that certain foods tend to decrease the frequency and severity of attacks. Foods that have shown some benefit include fresh fruits and vegetables, foods high in vitamins C and E and Omega 3's. The Mediterranean diet has also been named in various studies as helping to lessen the frequency and severity of chronic asthma. Maintaining a healthy weight and exercise can also help control chronic asthma.

Cancer
Cancer is a complicated disease to manage from many perspectives and can have a tremendous impact on an individual's life. Because there are so many forms of cancers and so many treatment modalities available depending on the type of cancer and the individual, the discussion here will be generalized and pertinent to the diagnosis as a whole.

Of course the best way to start a discussion about cancer is to address preventive measures such as; lifestyle choices, diet, weight management, avoiding exposures to cancer causing agents and regular disease screenings. Even when all of the right things are done, many people will fall victim to this devastating disease.

Once diagnosed with cancer, there are certain basics that everyone should do:

1. Ask for an English translation to what the health care provider just said. Chances are your health care provider will give you the text book name and you won't know what it is let alone where it is.

2. Ask for the staging of the cancer. This is a rating scale between 1 and 4. 1 being the earliest stage and 4 being a more advanced and aggressive stage.

3. Discuss treatment options with your health care provider and ask where the specialists for the type of cancer you are diagnosed with are located.

4. Go home and do credible research at the library, on line, with friends and family. Get specifics and check the validity of the resources.

5. Get a second opinion. Always get a second opinion, not only about the diagnosis but also the treatment options.

6. Be proactive and be a participant in your treatment and recovery. Put yourself in the best possible position to heal. If you didn't have a healthy lifestyle before the diagnosis, being diagnosed should give you some incentive. Research dietary changes eliminating as many preservatives as possible and increasing your intake of natural and organic foods.

7. Join a support group.

8.) Become active in activities sponsored by wellness centers, hospitals and clinics.

9. Do not fall victim to treatment scams and pie-in-the-sky promises.

10. Do not feel pressured by a health care provider to act before getting a second opinion. An exception would be certain life threatening situations.

11. Make sure that your medical-legal documents are up to date and that your legal affairs are in order. These should be up to date regardless, but depending on your diagnosis and prognosis, it may be worth a double check to make sure that your wishes are followed.

12. Have pertinent and meaningful conversations with friends and family. This is something that should be done as we journey through life, but if you haven't done this thus far you may find it beneficial. Keeping friends and family in the dark is generally not going to be helpful to you or them. This is a time in your life that you will need and want all the help and support that you can get.

13. Expect setbacks and have ideas on how to work through them.

14. Keep your life as normal as possible.

15. Maintain a positive mental attitude and reduce the stress in your life as much as possible. Stress makes any kind of healing more difficult.

16. Most importantly, put yourself first. Get plenty of rest, recruit help and learn how to set boundaries with family and friends when necessary.

It is much easier to say many of the above suggestions than it is to do them, especially when confronted with such a diagnosis. Yes, cancer can be deadly, but it can also be an opportunity for personal growth.

Colds

The common cold is one of the most stubborn disease processes known to mankind. It seems odd that in an era where medicine has made so many strides in disease management, that no one can really find a cure for the cold. There are however several ways to minimize your cold experiences.

The first step in keeping colds at bay is to keep your immune system strong and effective. To accomplish this, eat a well balanced diet, exercise, get adequate sleep and avoid antibiotics whenever possible. Having spent many years in an emergency room setting, I have seen a lot people coming to the ER for relief of cold symptoms, and many seeking antibiotic therapy to lessen the severity and length of the cold. Because colds are caused by viruses and not bacteria, antibiotics are a bad choice and do not help. Yes, once you start taking an antibiotic you may see an improvement in the symptoms, but that improvement would have occurred just as soon without the antibiotics. While antibiotics are fabulous drugs when used appropriately, when used inappropriately, the consequences can be significant. We have seen dramatic increases in the number of antibiotic resistant bacteria due to the inappropriate prescribing of antibiotics. Even when used appropriately, antibiotics destroy the normal flora in the body which is a huge part of the body's immune system and disease fighting abilities.

So why do health care providers prescribe antibiotics for people with colds? There are generally two main reasons. Number one, some health care providers are afraid of legal action. They fear that if it is a bacterial infection, and they don't treat it and the patient gets worse they could be guilty of malpractice down the road. So basically, they are working on the premise of better to be safe than sorry. The second reason is one that we discussed in earlier chapters, health care providers are in business, and when customers come in requesting something the health care providers want to keep their customers happy and give them what they ask for. Once again, as an advocate for yourself you have to take some responsibility in this area and have an honest discussion with your health care provider. If your health care provider tells you you have a cold and writes a prescription for an antibiotic, ask him why.

Instead of demanding antibiotics for cold symptoms, use over-the-counter fever reducers, cough medicines and/or decongestants. Be sure none of these medications interfere with other medications that you are taking, and read labels carefully to make sure the medications you are taking do not contain the same ingredients. Many of the over-the -counter medications will contain similar ingredients, and it is very easy to ingest high levels of the same medication which can lead to organ damage and other serious adverse reactions. For example, many of the decongestants contain stimulants and can put you at risk for fast or irregular heart rhythms. Many over-the-counter medications contain acetaminophen as a fever reducer. Taking more than one medication containing acetaminophen can cause serious liver damage. You may also consider using more natural methods such as; warm steam vaporizers, vaporubs, honey, tepid baths, etc. If you experience high fevers that don't come down with fever reducers, tepid baths, etc., and/or moderate to severe shortness of breath, a trip to the ER may be advised.

Of course, one of the easiest ways to avoid the cold bug is by practicing good hand hygiene. Washing your hands frequently, keeping your hands away from your face and sneezing and coughing into your sleeve will help reduce the spread of the cold virus. There are also several over-the-counter supplements that many people swear by. Zinc and Echinacea are two supplements that have been touted as having abilities to keep the immune system strong and to shorten the duration of cold-like symptoms. Other over-the-counter supplements combine the Zinc and Echinacea with high doses of vitamins, especially vitamins C and E. Keep in mind, if you are taking prescription medications, to check with your pharmacist or health care provider before taking any supplements to insure they do not interact with your prescription medications.

Depression
Depression is one of the most misdiagnosed diseases in health care.
Often times the diagnosis of depression is made when there are no
diagnostic criteria to support the diagnosis. Or, it is a diagnosis that is
missed when there is an overwhelming amount of diagnostic criteria
to support it, but it is overlooked. So, how can this happen? There are
several reasons why this happens. First, many of the criteria that
support the diagnosis of this disease process are subjective in nature
and are dependent not only on the patient's reporting, but also the
health care provider's interpretation. Secondly, many cases of depression are being diagnosed by practitioners in the medical realm instead
of the mental health realm. While many medical professionals are
trained to assess for depression, they have not had the concentrated
training of those in the mental health profession, thereby not always
applying the criteria to diagnose appropriately. The third reason
for misdiagnosis is astute marketing departments of pharmaceutical companies, and the many advertisements flashed before the
public for consumption. Once again, this leads to the patient going to
their health care provider and demanding a fix, and the health care
provider wanting to keep a happy customer. And the final reason is,
patients want to feel better and they want it fast. Dealing with depression whether it be acute or chronic, can be a time consuming process
that requires a concerted effort on the part of the patient, and unfortunately many patients don't want to work that hard or wait that long.
They want a quick fix, but unfortunately that is not always the right
answer.

Let's step back a minute and take a look at the two primary types of
depression. The first type of depression is chronic depression which
is a depressive state that lasts for more than six months. The second
type is acute depression which generally lasts less than six months.
Both types of depression can run the gamut from mild to severe.
Both types can also be caused by different factors such as situational,
chemical and/or hormonal imbalances, genetics, or substance abuse.
When deciding how to treat either type of depression, the patient and
the health care provider should take time to examine the causes of the
depression before deciding on a treatment protocol. There are cases

when lifestyle changes, counseling and patience are the best way to treat depression. Other times, prescription medications combined with lifestyle changes and counseling are the best choices. There is generally never just one treatment protocol that is successful in treating depression.

If you think that you and/or a loved are suffering from depression, it is best to ask your family health care provider for a referral to a mental health specialist. To truly diagnose any type or level of depression requires a thorough assessment by a professional who has had extensive training with the assessment tools, as well as the established diagnostic criteria. Unfortunately, patients will go to their doctors and tell them they are depressed and walk out with a prescription. This prescription medication will alter the patient's chemical/hormonal function which may not be warranted.

An example to illustrate this point comes from one of our clients who went to her daughter's doctor about one year following the death of her husband of 60 years. The doctor asked her if she was depressed. Her response was that no one had ever asked her that question before. She proceeded to state that she had noticed that she cried more easily than she had before. She also reported that she enjoyed life, exercised daily, socialized with friends and maintained her household independently. Because of her response, the doctor wrote her a prescription for an anti-depressant and sent her on her way. She called us several days later after reading about the medication on-line. She said, "I don't think there is anything wrong with my Serotonin levels, why do I need this?" Fortunately, this patient had a good insight into her mental and physical health. The patient was no doubt still suffering somewhat from the grief process of losing her husband of 60 years. It was okay for her to occasionally cry and to grieve her loss. This is an important part of the process of moving forward, and no amount of medication is going to fix it. The medication may mask the grief and can, in some circumstances, contribute to more problems, both physical and mental.

Now let's take a look at the other side of coin, another patient that experiences the same type of loss, but becomes isolated from friends, unable to maintain her household, loses interests in favorite activities, increases or decreases dietary intake, etc. This person may indeed meet the clinical criteria for depression. She has been unable to address the issues at hand as the result of the stress of the situation. Severe and prolonged stress and grieving can indeed have an impact on the body's chemical and hormonal balance, and counseling along with a medication regime may be appropriate. Does it then become a permanent condition? Not necessarily. It is possible at some point this patient may be able to be weaned gradually from the medication, as the mind and body start working together again.

Continuing to explore this continuum, we have a patient either because of situational circumstances, genetics, and/or chemical/hormonal imbalances that has, over the course of their lifetime, battled severe depression, been unable to maintain a job, been unable to maintain family and social relationships, and has had trouble functioning in everyday life. This patient may require a multifaceted approach that may follow her throughout her life span. If this condition is not properly diagnosed and treated, it can have dire consequences. Depression symptoms may also be due to life circumstances and may require behavioral or life changes verses a medication approach. A thorough assessment by a professional can help determine whether or not your type of depression is clinical in nature or situational.

The moral of the story is, depression is a complex disease process and should not be taken lightly, nor should it be treated without thought and attention to detail by a combination of medical and mental health professionals. As with other medications, antidepressants are not just a panacea to be passed out without consideration. These medications can be a great adjunct to a well-balanced care plan, but given to the wrong people for the wrong reasons can have some incredible and unwanted side effects. In some people, antidepressants can increase the risk of suicidal ideation, suicide and increased depression. Make sure that before asking your health care provider for a prescription or

taking a prescription without a thorough multi-disciplinary assessment, that you thoroughly understand the risks and benefits of all
options and treatment protocols.

Diabetes

Diabetes is a complex disease and often difficult to manage. There are
two primary types of diabetes, Type I and Type II. Type I diabetes is
sometimes referred to as juvenile onset diabetes and diagnosed early
in life. This type of diabetes is also sometimes called insulin dependent diabetes, meaning that the only way to treat it is with insulin
injections. Type II diabetes is generally seen later in life and is usually
a result of lifestyle choices, but can also have a genetic predisposition component. In severe cases of Type II diabetes or cases that have
progressed over time, it may become necessary to treat with insulin
injections, thereby also becoming insulin dependent.

While Type I diabetes is not preventable, the managing of this disease
process can usually be impacted by lifestyle choices. Compliance, or
lack thereof, is often a problem in Type I diabetes. Watching dietary
intake and monitoring blood sugar levels is imperative in the control
of diabetes. Without consistent compliance, Type I diabetes can have a
devastating effect on all organ systems of the body. Even with compliance, the impact of diabetes can be troublesome at best. To minimize
this impact, work closely with your health care provider in gaining
control of the disease process. Monitor blood levels closely, keep accurate records of successes and failures and discuss new advances in
treatments with your health care provider.

Diabetes is an area where there is great opportunity for you to advocate for advancements in the treatment of this disease. There are
many new areas of research involving stem cells and skin cells which
are being touted as a potential cure for diabetes. As an advocate for
yourself or loved one, it is advisable to read about these new developments and how they will impact the management of this disease and
then get involved. There of course have been many ethical debates
about stem cell research, so it is important for you to keep your ethical
beliefs in mind and the various methods used to harvest stem cells.

Advocating for yourself and loved ones is a huge responsibility so make sure that you have all the facts and then start advocating.

Type II diabetes can be just as impactful as Type I, but there can be more of a lifestyle component involved. In some mild cases of Type II diabetes, maintaining a healthy weight and diet control can sometimes reverse the process. Every day we see patients who have lost weight by changing their eating and exercise habits and have been able to control their diabetes by this means, instead of relying on medication control. If you should decide to undertake lifestyle changes, make sure that you work closely with your health care provider. Do not stop taking your medication unless advised to do so after close monitoring and discussion with your health care provider. When Type II diabetes is caused more by genetic factors, it may be less likely to achieve a reversal by the above mentioned means, but you can still lessen the impact of the disease process. Either way, never stop taking your medication without a discussion with your health care provider. We have unfortunately seen a lot of patients who, after taking their medications for a while and getting control of their blood sugar levels, have stopped the medications because their blood sugar levels have normalized. Keep in mind, the medications are why the levels have normalized and stopping them abruptly can lead to serious health consequences.

Emergency room usage
While not a disease classification, emergency room usage can play a huge role in disease management. It is also an area where you, as a patient, can advocate for yourself and others by ensuring that your use of emergency services is appropriate.

It is unfortunate, but there are a lot of people who use emergency rooms as their primary physician. Sometimes this is because of insurance issues such as lack of health insurance. Other times it is a result of impatience and wanting to be seen now. When patients use the emergency room in the wrong way, it can often lead to lapses in care, inadequate disease management, poor follow through, misdiagnosis and exposure to infectious diseases. The other major issue is the overcrowding of the nation's emergency rooms, which hampers their ability to deal with true life threatening emergencies and crisis situations.

Solving the problems of inappropriate emergency room usage will not be an easy task. It will take a multi-pronged approach, including some major reform of our health care system, consistent and constant educational programs and individual, personal responsibility. Denying someone care because they don't have insurance, is not a viable or humane option. Free clinics and governmental health care programs are already overwhelmed, so even if the uninsured try to use other services they are often turned away. Solving many of these issues will take many years and are much more complex than can be dealt with in this arena. We can look at some of the areas that just about every health care consumer can participate in, and those areas include; personal choice and responsibility, paying attention to current trends and advocating for appropriate reform.

Let's take a look at how we, as individuals, can most appropriately use emergency room services. When possible, maintain health insurance coverage. Find a primary health care provider that you feel confident and comfortable with and stay with her. Follow sound health prevention and maintenance programs. Utilize sound judgment when deciding when and how to use emergency services. Unfortunately, there are a lot of patients who see the emergency room as a convenient and immediate solution to non-emergent problems. These patients are putting themselves at increased risk when they use the emergency room for non-emergent purposes. Keep in mind what happens in emergency rooms. People with various infectious processes come there for treatment. The emergency room can also be a place of high drama and emotion that can sometimes turn violent. In other words, it is possible to leave an emergency room in worse shape than when you arrived. Prior to using emergency services ask yourself the following questions:

1. Do I feel that my condition is of a life threatening nature?

2. Can I safely wait until I can see my regular health care provider?

3. Have I tried comfort measures that have failed?

4. Can my problem be treated at a clinic or urgent care?

5. Is my condition serious enough to call for emergency transport?

Many times, asking these questions will help prevent an unnecessary visit to the ER. Let's take a look at some of the conditions or scenarios that would generally be valid reasons to use emergency services.

1. Fevers greater than 103 degrees that are not relieved with over-the-counter fever reducers.

2. Chest pain accompanied by radiating pain, nausea/vomiting, weakness, shortness of breath, gray/pallor coloring of the skin, dizziness, severely increased or decreased blood pressure and/or pulse.

3. The worst headache of your life that is untouched by over-the-counter medications.

4. Traumatic head injuries.

5. Numbness, tingling, vision changes, slurred speech, memory problems, facial drooping, and loss of use of extremities.

6. Moderate to severe abdominal pain with a rapid onset, with or without associated nausea/vomiting, diarrhea, inability to urinate and/or defecate, bloody urine, stool or vomit.

7. Broken bones.

8. Blood pressures over 200/100.

9. Rapid pulse.

10. Difficulty breathing.

11. Suicidal or homicidal ideations.

12. Intentional or unintentional overdoses or ingestions.

13. Severe eye injuries.

14. Throat swelling with inability to swallow saliva, choking or difficulty breathing.

15. Lacerations.

16. Nose bleeds that last more than 15 minutes despite continuous pressure.

17. Vaginal bleeding where you are soaking one or more pads an hour for more than three hours.

18. Moderate to severe allergic reactions.

19. Intense, sudden onset of unexplained pain.

20. Rapidly appearing skin infections with associated redness, swelling, heat, red streaks, discharge/drainage, and foul odor.

21. Rashes associated with severe headache, neck stiffness, high fever and lethargy.

22. Severe alcohol intoxication.

23. Severe heat or cold exposure.

24. Severe sunburn with severe blistering and multiple skin layer damage.

25. Burns

26. Chemical and environmental exposures.

27. Carbon monoxide poisoning.

28. Severe dehydration.

29. Sickle cell crisis.

30. Severe pain associated with malignancies.

31. Moderate to severe motor vehicle accidents.

32. Gunshot and stab wounds.

33. Extremely high or low blood sugar readings.

Now let's take a look at some of the reasons not to use emergency services but to treat at home or visit your primary health care provider, urgent care or clinic:

1. Chapped lips. (Sad but true, we see it frequently.)

2. Minor to moderate sunburns.

3. Razor rash on the legs. (This one came in by ambulance.)

4. Colds and flu without associated difficulty breathing.

5. Hangovers.

6. Minor to moderate nausea/vomiting, diarrhea associated with simple food poisoning or stomach viruses lasting less than 48 hours.

7. Sprains

8. Minor scrapes, abrasions, lacerations without gaping cuts.

9. Chronic pain conditions.

10. Mild to moderate headaches.

11. Minor motor vehicle accidents.

12. Pregnancy tests.

13. Medication refills.

14. Minor rashes/allergic reactions.

15. Sexually transmitted disease testing.

16. Minor sore throats and earaches.

17. Minor urinary tract infections.

18. Borderline hypertension.

19. Abnormal vaginal bleeding where bleeding is not heavy as described above.

20. Low grade fevers or fevers that respond to over-the-counter treatments.

21. Lumps, bumps and pains that have been present for more than six months.

22. Routine disease management.

23. Stubbed toes without deformity.

While these lists are not all inclusive, they should serve as a guide to appropriate usage of emergency services. It is up to each individual to advocate and assume responsibility for how these services are used. Without personal and individual responsibility, these services will continue to be challenged. The more these services are stretched and challenged, the more patient safety will be put in jeopardy.

Gallbladder Disease
The gallbladder is such a small part of the anatomy, yet can cause some huge problems. As with so many things, gallbladder disease can be influenced by both lifestyle choices and genetics. The one life style choice that can have the biggest impact on the health and longevity of your gallbladder, is a diet high in fatty foods.

The gallbladder produces a substance called bile which is released into the intestinal system to aid in digestion. When you have a diet high in fat it, in simple terms, can over overwhelm the gallbladder causing a development of gall stones. Many times, gall stones can hang out in the gallbladder and never cause a problem. Other times, those stones can move and drop into the gallbladder's duct, blocking the release of bile into the intestinal system. When this happens, there is generally a great deal of pain in the right upper abdominal area and back area along with occasional nausea and vomiting. Sometimes, these stones will move out of the duct and be flushed from the body. Generally, when this happens once, it will happen again. Because of the severity of discomfort and/or frequency of the sequence, surgery is indicated to remove the gallbladder. In some instances, even when the gallbladder is removed, the stones will remained lodged in the duct which can cause severe pain, nausea, vomiting, and fever. When the symptoms become this severe, it is indicative of a total blockage leading to a backflow of bile into the pancreas. This can lead to pancreatitis and, in severe cases, can lead to life-threatening situations. If you should experience the severe range of these symptoms, a trip to the emergency room is warranted.

The good news is that you can lower your risk of gallbladder disease by watching the fat content in your diet. The other good news is you can live without the gallbladder. After the gallbladder is removed, the bile goes from the liver directly into the intestinal tract. After surgery, some people will experience increased instances of diarrhea and nausea. These symptoms are generally temporary, but some patients have reported increased food sensitivities after gallbladder removal. So what should you do if your health care provider tells you that you have gallbladder disease?

1. As stated earlier, many people live with gallstones in their gallbladder without them causing any problems. Occasionally, you will have some sort of testing done, and the gallstone will be discovered. If this is the case and you are not experiencing any symptoms, then you probably don't need to consider surgery.

2. If you do experience a gallbladder attack, depending on the severity, you may want to take a wait and see approach. There are some cleanses and treatments that some people have reported success with. Trying these treatments to rid the gallbladder of stones, may be worth trying before going under the knife.

3. If, after every time you eat, you experience right upper quadrant abdominal pain, gastric reflux, shoulder/back pain and nausea/vomiting, you will probably want to talk to your health care provider about a referral to a surgeon. (See earlier and later discussions on surgeries to know what to ask.)

4. Once surgery has been decided upon, the decision of how the surgery will be done will be the next concern. Most surgeons will remove the gallbladder laparoscopically. They will cut several very small incisions in which to insert the surgical tools and remove the gallbladder through one of the small holes. The other option is an open surgery, where the surgeon will cut about a 4 to 5 inch long incision and remove the gallbladder that way. The third option may be a combination of both. Occasionally, a surgeon will start the surgery laparoscopically and find other complications such as

infection, inflammation or tumors that require they then proceed
through an open procedure. The risk for this third option increases
if you have had a number of other abdominal surgeries or procedures and have a buildup of adhesions or scar tissue. Of course,
laparoscopic surgery generally results in less post-operative pain
and quicker recovery times and is the preferred method when there
is a choice.

While most people will have very few, if any, problems after this type
of surgery, some may start having the same type of symptoms again.
This is generally the result of gallstones getting caught in the common
bile duct. This typically requires an intervention called an ERCP,
where a gastrointestinal doctor will go in with a scope and remove
the stone. On rare occasions, the problem can be the result of a tumor
in the area. Either way, you should make sure to follow up with your
health care provider to prevent future complications.

Heart Disease
Heart disease is a very complex disease with many processes. In the
medical world, heart disease can also be called cardiovascular disease
(CVD) and/or coronary artery disease (CAD). Sometimes these terms
are used interchangeably and other times there are differences in the
processes and the outcomes. For the purpose of this book, we will cover
this vital, yet involved, disease with a rather general approach.

Family history is probably one of the most predictive factors of heart
disease. That being said, if you know that you have a strong family
history, lifestyle choices and regular monitoring of your heart health
can change the trend in your family. Lifestyle choices, while not
always easy, are more in your control than the genetics you came with.
Your genetics are not a life sentence, but a push to being proactive
in your health care choices. Below we will discuss some of the more
common heart related diagnoses and ways in which you can advocate
for yourself throughout the process.

1. Cholesterol is one of the main causes of heart disease and many
   health care providers are screening their patients routinely to

ascertain these levels. When the good cholesterol is down and the bad cholesterol is up, your health care provider may want to prescribe a medication to get the levels in line. Once again, keep in mind that all medications come with side effects. The most common side effect of some of the cholesterol medications is muscle and joint pain. Many people find this almost debilitating. There are other choices and if you experience this side effect, talk to your health care provider about other options.

One option is making dietary, exercise and lifestyle choices. The second option is talking with your physician about natural alternatives. Many traditional health care providers will not be particularly well informed on natural alternatives. There are many reasons for this lack of knowledge. Some alternative treatments have not been extensively researched and there is little scientific evidence to back up the claims. Health care providers are uncomfortable recommending these alternatives out of fear of being accused of not practicing within the standards of care. Secondly, many of the alternative choices are not regulated by any regulatory agency which raises questions about content and quality. Lastly, going alternative is not as profitable for the traditional health care provider. Keep in mind, that lifestyle changes and alternative therapies may not be enough if your cholesterol levels are being genetically driven. Often medications are the only way to bring the levels back in line.

If discussing alternative therapies with your health care provider, make sure that you have done your research on the therapies. Make sure the resources are unbiased and not profiting from the sales of such therapies. Be wary of practitioners that are selling alternative therapies as part of their practice. Talk to your local pharmacist on the safety of utilizing alternative therapies with other medications you are taking and your personal health history.

2. Chest Pain- Chest pain is the number one symptom associated with heart disease. Oftentimes, chest pain is one of the last symptoms to present. There are many people who suffer from heart disease who

never experience chest pain. While chest pain is often associated
with heart attacks, there are many other causes of chest pain such
as: pulled/strained chest wall muscles, blood clots in the lungs,
pneumonia, stress and anxiety, gastric reflux disease (heartburn),
hemothorax/pneumothorax (blood/air leaks around the lungs),
tumors and musculoskeletal issues.

So how do you know if your chest pain is being caused by your
heart? Many times it is not easy and it is the one thing that when
in doubt, it is best to get it checked sooner rather than later. As a
rule, pain that occurs with movement or worsened by certain move-
ments is most commonly associated with muscle strain. A burning
sensation after eating usually is caused by reflux of stomach acids.
The other causes of chest pain listed above are a little bit harder to
distinguish from cardiac pain, but are also reasons to seek attention. Most cardiac related chest pain occurs with activity and/or
stress, is relieved with rest, radiates to jaws, neck, back and either
arm. It also is usually associated with shortness of breath, sweating
and occasionally nausea and vomiting. In women, the signs can be
much more subtle and are often missed as being cardiac related
even by many health care providers. Women often experience more
abdominal related symptoms such as abdominal pain, nausea,
vomiting, dizziness or extreme tiredness. A lot of women may think
that they have food poisoning, heartburn or gallbladder disease and
delay seeking treatment.

The most important thing to remember when experiencing chest
pain is that time equals muscle. In other words, the longer you
wait to seek treatment for cardiac related chest pain, the more
heart muscle is at risk for damage. If you experience more subtle
symptoms such as increased tiredness, frequent stomach upset and
shortness of breath with mild exertion, it is best to see your health
care provider to prevent a possible catastrophic event.

So, you are not sure what is causing the pain, but you are
concerned that it might be your heart. The latest recommendations are to take an aspirin and go to your doctor, urgent care or

emergency room, preferably with someone else driving or by emergency transport. When taking an aspirin for chest pain, it is most advisable to take 4 baby aspirin or one 325 mg aspirin. Chewing the aspirin has been reported to work the quickest, but if you can't stand the thought of chewing the aspirin, go ahead and take it with water. There are times when aspirin is contraindicated such as with a severe allergy to aspirin or asthma. Many people who suffer from peptic ulcer disease or severe reflux disease will hesitate to take the aspirin, because they have been advised not to take aspirin due to an increased risk of stomach bleeding. If you suspect that you are in the midst of a cardiac event, the benefits of the aspirin outweigh the risks of stomach issues.

3. Cardiac testing – There are several tests that can be done to monitor the state of your heart's health. Some tests are non-invasive and inexpensive; others are more invasive, more expensive and come with higher risks. It is important to discuss the risks and benefits of each test with your health care provider. If your health care provider has a high degree of suspicion of heart disease, he may order a progressive series of tests to make sure. Of course, some tests are more telling than others. EKG's, one of the most common tests ordered to initially test the condition of the heart, are not always able to detect changes that can lead to a serious cardiac event. As a matter of fact, about a third of the people coming to the emergency room for chest pain have normal EKGs, but they are actually in the midst of a heart attack. In this case, the health care provider may order a series of blood tests to check for enzymes that are released into the blood system when heart muscle is being damaged. These tests are also not always conclusive, and the doctor may want you stay overnight to have the tests redrawn every six hours to make sure that these levels are not changing over time. If you have several risks factors for heart disease, it is best to heed your health care provider's advice and stay for additional testing.

4. Silent Heart Attacks – Thus far, we have discussed the very outward symptoms of heart disease, but it is possible to have a heart attack and not know it. This is of particular concern to

diabetics who may have nerve damage caused by diabetes that affects the ability of the patient to feel the pain. Other times, it is possible that the symptoms mimic other things that don't concern the patient enough to seek help, and they go about their business not knowing that they have suffered such an event. Generally, silent heart attacks are relatively minor events, but can be a sign of bigger things to come. Sometimes a patient will show EKG changes during a screening EKG. Depending on age, risk factors and medical history, the doctor may order additional testing to help diagnose underlying problems. Even though silent heart attacks are generally mild, there is usually some associated heart muscle damage. In some cases, the heart will develop what they call collateral circulation which is, in simple terms, the blood in the heart finding alternate routes. Many people can actually do very well with this type of circulation and, depending on other factors; a health care provider may decide not to treat, if the collateral circulation is working for the heart muscle and the patient.

5. Abnormal Heart Rhythms- Rhythms that are too fast, too slow, flip-flopping, skipping beats, or creating extra beats can be an indication that something is disrupting your normal heart function. Some of these rhythms are generally nothing to worry about, but some are signs that are warning you that something is very wrong. When trying to decide if abnormal heart rhythms are something to be concerned about, ask yourself several questions. Is it associated with pain? Is it a result of something you did or are doing? Are you having other symptoms such as shortness of breath, feeling light headed or faint, and/or anxious? If the answers to any of the questions are yes, it is advisable to get it checked. Let's look at some of the different types of heart rhythms and some of the causes.

Rapid Heart Rate- The normal range for heart rate is 60-100 beats per minute (bpm). Heart rates greater than 100bpm can be the result of many things such as caffeine intake, sugar intake, fevers, exercise, illness, anxiety, stress, over-the-counter drugs like decongestants that often contain stimulants, diet products, being in poor physical condition, alcohol, dehydration, illicit drugs, prescriptions drugs, electrolyte imbalances, hormonal imbalances and the list goes on. Many of these things are not serious in nature and can be corrected by watching what you eat, drink and take. Others require examination by a health care provider, or in severe cases, a trip to the ER. You should be concerned when the heart stays elevated over a period of time, is extremely elevated over 120 beats per minute (without physical exertion), or when you experience symptoms such as pain, shortness of breath, dizziness, etc. Heart rates over 140 beats per minute should be considered an urgent situation and treated immediately by emergency personnel.

Slow Heart Rate- Heart rates below 60bpm usually are benign and often found in people who are physically fit. Other times, slow heart rates can be caused by blockages or disruptions in the heart muscle's electrical circuits. Slow heart rates caused by these disruptions should be evaluated by your health care provider. If you are experiencing lethargy, dizziness, pain and/or confusion, it would once again be considered an emergent situation.

Dropped Beats/Extra Beats – These also are often benign and can be traced to dietary intake, activity and/or medications, etc. If you experience these irregular beats for an extended period of time or experience symptoms, they certainly should be evaluated to rule out other causes.

Obviously, this is a very cursory overview of heart disease. It is a disease process that requires a close relationship with a health care provider that you trust, compliance in treatment and medication regimes and, of course, lifestyle changes. While heart disease can be a life threatening condition, it can often be managed, but should never be ignored.

Obesity
Obesity has become the latest and perhaps one of the biggest health epidemics in the United States. The causes of obesity are both

numerous and complex. Many health care providers and politicians are proposing many solutions to get the problem under control. We have heard about the proposals to remove certain ingredients from our food supplies, removing items from vending machines at schools and businesses and eliminating certain types of food from the shelves. Some argue that these proposals are government interference in our personal choices; others argue that everyone has to pay for someone else's bad dietary choices. Regardless of which side of the argument you are on, the problem is huge, and the first step is education. Education certainly isn't going to solve the problem, but it is perhaps the most unobtrusive choice we have that protects our rights as citizens and cuts our costs in dealing with this epidemic.

How did we get here? Technology can probably be blamed for many of the things that have led to this epidemic. Plows are no longer pushed through the fields, water does not have to be hauled and food is not something that we have to chase or grow ourselves. Since we no longer have to perform these back breaking tasks for survival, we have to now schedule time in our day to do something that resembles back breaking work. The food is not rationed by what we can grow or catch, but how much we can afford and how quickly we can get it. It is easy to go to the stores, restaurants, and fast food establishments and find lots of things to eat without working for them in the traditional sense. But gee, isn't it nice that we have all these choices and conveniences? Now we just have to learn how to have them and remain healthy. Fortunately, through increased education and awareness, there has been an increase in knowledge of healthier alternatives and choices. It took us a long time to get here and it no doubt is going to take us a long time to get back to some sort of balance.

Until we find a balance and decrease the causes of obesity in our country, we have to look at ways to treat it as a disease process. There certainly is not a shortage of diet books, exercise books and videos, health clubs and treatments, but which one is going to be best for you? As an advocate for yourself, this is going to be a decision that requires extensive education and discipline. If obesity is a problem for you or a loved one, and it's time for a change, examine all of your options carefully. Below we will cover some of the most common and/ or popular treatments for obesity and their risks and benefits. Which option will be the right one for you, will be a decision that you should make after examining all of the choices, talking with health care providers in both the medical and mental health realms, examining your own medical history and the risks and benefits of each method of obesity treatment.

1. Diet and Exercise – Diet and exercise is certainly the most natural method of weight loss as long as you make the right choices, and make it a permanent part of your overall health care approach. The diet you choose should not be a fad, but a sustainable and healthy balance that you can maintain and manage over the life span. An exercise program should start out slowly and also be something that you can incorporate into your lifestyle. The benefits of choosing the right diet and exercise program are mostly positive when it is something that can be maintained over the long haul. The risk of undertaking this option is, if you pick an unbalanced plan or get too carried away with your exercise regime, it may lead to injury and joint problems.

It seems so easy to say that diet and exercise can cure you of obesity, but it is a huge challenge for most obese people. If it were easy, we wouldn't be having this discussion. Prior to taking on this challenge, it is important to try to figure out how you got to the obese level. This requires a great deal of introspection into why you eat the way you do and why you make the choices that you do. Ask yourself if it is because of depression, a significant life event, your lifestyle, the people that you surround yourself with and/or your self esteem or self image. Sometimes it is helpful to get outside help to find the answers. Support groups, mental health counselors and even friends and family can help you find those answers. Once you find the answers to why you make the choices that you do, the easier it will be to address and change them.

2. Medications – There are times when obesity can be traced to imbalances in the body. Thyroid imbalances are generally the most common ones found in obesity, but there can be many other chemical and hormonal imbalances. A thorough physical and lab work up through your primary health care provider can help uncover these imbalances. Certain abnormalities will require a medication regime to get back into balance; others can be corrected better with dietary and lifestyle changes. Make sure that you have a detailed discussion with your health care provider as to what is the best and most natural way to get your body back into balance.

Of course, a lot of people will go to the grocery store, pharmacy and/or health food store to find an over-the-counter medication that will promote weight loss. This solution to solve an obesity problem is generally ineffective and many times dangerous or life threatening.

Many of the over-the-counter dietary supplements contain high doses of stimulants. It would not be a good idea for a person whose cardiovascular system is already being stressed by obesity to take a stimulant on top of it. Many of these drugs can cause problems even for young people who still have a rather healthy and strong cardiovascular system. Not only do these drugs stress the heart, but they can also cause mental health issues such as anxiety, panic and hallucinations. Keep in mind that most dietary supplements sold over-the-counter in this country are not regulated and knowing the exact content of these medications is almost impossible. While there has been some improvement in the truth in labeling, the problem is that it can be years after these medications hit the market before someone catches a labeling problem. When advocating for yourself, it is best to avoid over-the-counter weight loss supplements.

The other choices in weight loss medications are the prescription medications that you can get through your health care provider. There are several different types of medication on the market at this time. Many of these medications work by either changing how the body absorbs fats and/or by altering the way your body produces certain chemicals that affect hunger or satiety responses in the body. For some people, this is a viable alternative and is a way to jump start a weight loss program that can be closely monitored by their primary health care provider. Even with the prescription weight loss medications, a change in dietary intake and exercise is necessary to achieve maximum effectiveness. One word of caution with the prescription weight loss medications, they are still relatively new on the market and their long term effects may not yet be known. While most prescription medications go through a fairly thorough review by the Food and Drug Administration, many of the long term effects are not discovered until the drug has been on the market for several years and has been available to a wide cross section of the population.

3. Surgery – Over the last several decades, surgery to reduce the size of the stomach has become a popular method of weight loss management. The two primary surgeries are the gastric bypass and the lap-band procedures. There has been controversy and disagreement over the overall benefits and effectiveness of these procedures. Initially, these procedures were developed to treat the severely obese. The typical patient was generally someone who was at an immediate risk for serious health consequences and/or was so obese that exercise was thought to be impossible or too risky. Also in the beginning, the patients were required to be at least 100 pounds overweight and were to have gone through at least a year of nutritional, weight loss and psychological counseling prior to being approved for the surgery. Some of these restrictions were guided by the insurance industry and others by the medical profession. More recently some of these requirements have been eased, or health care professionals have learned to skirt around some of the requirements creating more

controversy and debate. Recently, there has been an increase in the number of these procedures. Some say this increase is in direct proportion to the increase in obesity, others say the surgery is being used as an alternative to lifestyle changes by those with mild to moderate obesity. Regardless of the controversy, there are important considerations to keep in mind when deciding which alternative is right for you.

First, let's look at the different ways that the surgery is accomplished. One of the first techniques of gastric surgery was the gastric stapling. In simple terms, the surgeon would go in and literally staple parts of the stomach together shrinking the stomach's capacity. This surgery worked well for many people initially, and especially for those patients who would stop eating when feeling satiated. The problem was that the stomach muscles can keep expanding, and the staples would come undone. So as patients adapted to the smaller stomach, they gradually started putting larger and larger quantities of food in their stomach, not realizing their stomachs were once again expanding, and the weight was adding up once again.

The next advancement in gastric surgery was the bypass surgery. This was a similar concept to the stapling except that instead of the stomach basically being halved, it is now being sectioned into 4 equal parts and the digestion is bypassed directly into the small intestine. The surgeon and the technique that the surgeon uses, dictates the level of success with this surgery. There is an area in the stomach where the muscle tissue is less pliable therefore less likely to expand and allow increased intake and regaining of the weight. If the surgeon bypasses in this area the success rate may be higher. Regardless of the location, it is still possible to re-stretch the stomach and regain the weight.

The latest development in gastric surgery is the Lap-band surgery. This is a surgery where the surgeon inserts a band around the stomach that can be tightened or loosened to achieve the best results and comfort level for the patient. This procedure is the easiest one to reverse. The disadvantage of this procedure is that many patients can't tolerate the symptoms of quicker stomach filling and will request the band be loosened. This is not always a bad thing, but weight loss will be slowed and, as in the other methods, weight may be regained.

The best way to benefit most from gastric surgery is to make sure that you go through all the preparatory steps such as psychological counseling to determine why you have a weight problem, nutritional counseling to learn how to prepare foods in a healthier way, exercise training to incorporate activity and cardiac benefits and, of course, a thorough medical exam to see if there are other causes leading to obesity. These steps seem to be no brainers, but in actuality a lot of patients never take any of these steps prior to undergoing the knife. Some surgeons are very good about insisting on these steps, but others aren't. Think about it, a surgeon whose livelihood depends on performing these surgeries is not going to want to wait for all of his patients to go through these steps. He makes more money by doing more surgeries. He may ask his patients if they have taken these steps, but then does nothing to insure that the recommended steps have been followed. Unfortunately, most patients don't want to wait, they have made the decision to have the surgery and they want to get on with it. When the proper steps are not followed, the chances of regaining the weight increase greatly.

The advantages of these surgical procedures can be numerous. For some people it can be a lifesaving measure. Many disease processes such as diabetes, hypertension, and cardiac problems can either be reversed or slowed by the tremendous weight loss that generally follows the procedures. Joint health can be enhanced by the reduction of weight. Self esteem, self image, anxiety and depression can also be aided by the weight loss for many people. The other advantage is that patients are able to sometimes lower their health care costs, increase their earning potential and experience activities that they may not have been able to experience while obese.

There can also be several disadvantages or risks associated with these procedures. With any surgery there are risks of infection, surgical complications, scar tissue, adhesions (tissue bands that adhere to internal muscles and organs), and in the worst case scenario, death. With gastric bypass, the absorption of vitamins and minerals is negatively impacted which can result in deficiencies such as anemia caused by lack of iron absorption. Prescription medication absorption can also be altered which can lead to adverse reactions and intolerance to certain medications, and you may develop a wide array of food intolerances. Many patients after gastric surgery find that some foods will make them violently ill or will get lodged in the stomach causing pain, nausea and vomiting. Most gastric patients need to be careful with sugar and caffeine intake as these substances will also absorb differently resulting in feelings of rapid heart rates and anxiety. These side effects are not all bad, in that, it does help the patient restrict her intake of some of the foods that are not that great for her in the first place, but it does take some time and trial and error before the patient will know what foods to avoid and what foods she can tolerate.

Alcohol becomes a problem for many patients after gastric surgery for a couple of reasons. First, alcohol is absorbed much more quickly resulting in quicker intoxication. Secondly, for those patients who had addictions to food, this addictive tendency often gets transferred to alcohol consumption. Another disadvantage in rapid weight loss that is not combined with some sort of exercise is a loss of skin tone resulting in sagging skin. Many patients find this negatively impacts their body image. This problem can be resolved through cosmetic surgery, but keep in mind that many insurance companies will not pay for this. Make sure that you check your insurance coverage and/or costs of the cosmetic surgeries prior to undergoing the gastric bypass.

Not all of the disadvantages are physical. Many disadvantages come in the psychological realm. Without proper counseling prior to surgery, you can find yourself gaining the weight back, because you have not dealt with the emotional issues that often surround obesity. The other thing that can happen, results from the psychological and emotional issues surrounding the weight loss and body image. Post-gastric surgery patients often find that after surgery they get different types of attention than they received when obese. They also experience a kind of a rebirth that can often lead to increased risk taking behavior and changes in interpersonal relationships.

When contemplating a weight loss plan and which direction you want to pursue, be sure to follow the recommended procedures, know the risks and benefits of each method and make sure that your physician is also following the recommended procedures. Don't fall victim to the latest fads; make changes that you are going to be able to incorporate into your lifestyle for the rest of your life.

Pain

Pain is a complicated process to manage for both patients and health care providers. There are basically two categories of pain that patients may experience throughout their life. Acute pain is something that all of us will probably experience at least once in our life and perhaps many times throughout the lifespan. Acute pain lasts for less than six months. It can occur with injury and/or a disease process. Acute pain can come and go and often be remedied with over-the-counter treatments, cold treatments or heat treatments. Occasionally, in the case of a more severe injury or surgery, stronger pain relief methods such as narcotics may be required. The treatment of acute pain can be accomplished quite easily through medical management and time. It is important to treat the pain in order to allow the body time to heal. For the treatment of acute pain, work with your health care provider to find the treatment that works best for you.

Often with acute pain treatment, your health care provider will try a combination of treatments to alleviate the pain such as prescription anti-inflammatories, narcotics, physical therapy and homeopathic remedies. Your health care provider will probably ask you to rate your pain on a 0-10 scale with 0 being no pain and 10 being the worst pain that you can imagine. Every patient is different in their tolerance and rating of pain. One patient may find that a broken toe ranks 5/10 while another patient may rate it 10/10. Which patient is right? They both are, because pain rating is subjective. Your health care provider should treat your pain based on your own personal perception of the pain. It is also important for the patient to realize that regardless of the pain treatment, all of the pain may not be completely relieved. The goal is to get the pain to where you, as an individual, can tolerate it and function. To manage acute pain most successfully, work closely with your health care provider, and not only take the medications prescribed or recommended, but also follow the treatment recommendations such as resting, icing, compressing and elevating the injured part.

Pain is a good sign that there is something wrong in the body and should be evaluated by a health care provider. Of course, if you spent the day chopping wood, you could bet that may be the cause of your pain. Usually over-the-counter medications and rest will solve that problem. If you cannot correlate the pain to something you did that may have caused it and it is not relieved by home based treatments, then by all means have it evaluated. Ignoring pain that lasts more than a couple of days is begging for trouble. While pain can be caused by too much activity, it can also be caused by inactivity. If you sit in the same position too long, lie for long periods of time on the same body part, etc. then try moving more frequently to see if the pain is relieved by increased circulation to the area. Pain can also be a result of psychological and emotional issues. If you suspect that your pain may be a result of an emotional issue, then talk to your health care provider for an appropriate referral to a mental health professional.

Because pain is so subjective in nature, it is often difficult for a health care provider to accurately diagnose the cause. If you feel that your health care provider is not paying attention to your complaints and you fear the pain is something of a more serious nature, explain this fear to your health care provider. Many patients have very good instincts or intuition about their bodies and it is important that you and your health care provider are on the same page. If your health care provider is not taking your complaints seriously, perhaps it is time to find another provider or at least get a second opinion.

The second type of pain is chronic pain. Chronic pain is generally a type of pain that lasts for longer than six months or, at times, can be a lifelong affliction. Chronic pain is even more of a challenge for both patients and health care providers. There are many things that can cause chronic pain including a previous trauma, injury and/or disease processes. Patients with chronic pain often get frustrated with their health care providers. They often feel that their providers are not taking them seriously or treating them appropriately. They also start to feel that they are being labeled a drug seeker. Health care providers get frustrated, because it is difficult to find a successful treatment plan for patients with chronic pain. Providers also can find themselves questioning drug seeking behavior and will recommend ineffective treatment modalities as a result. The patient-provider relationship then often takes a very confrontational turn.

The fact of the matter is that unfortunately there are a number of patients who are drug seeking and doctor shopping. Many times, this is a result of an inattentive health care provider who goes along only prescribing addictive pain treatments and not seeking alternative forms of treatment. When this happens, a patient's tolerance will increase and his dependence on the medications increases as well. When the doctor then starts to realize the severity of the problem, she cuts the patient off cold turkey and may not address the addiction issue. The patient also will not want to be cut off cold turkey and starts to find other sources for the medications. In order to treat chronic pain effectively, it is important for both the patient and the health care provider to have open and honest communication regarding addiction issues and alternative treatment regimes.

The best way to deal with chronic pain is to work closely with a health care provider who has experience in the type of pain that you are experiencing. Many times, family practitioners may not be able to keep up to date on dealing with certain types of chronic pain. You should have your family health care provider recommend a competent and reputable pain specialist who will work with your family practitioner in designing a pain control plan that can keep your chronic pain under control while lessening your chances of developing addiction issues.

If you or a loved one has already developed an addiction issue as the result of chronic pain, then the process becomes even more complicated, but not hopeless. First, you have to find alternative pain treatments by getting in touch with a legitimate pain specialist in your area and then find a good substance abuse treatment program. With this combination of health care providers, you can hopefully get both problems under control. Of course, the first step is to know and then to admit that a problem exists. If you are addicted, it may be difficult to see what has happened. When dealing with a loved one with an addiction problem, the challenge is getting her to see the problem. So how do you know if there is a problem? Ask several of the questions below; if the answers to most of them are yes, then it is time to seek help.

1. Does the pain seem to keep increasing despite higher doses of pain medications?

2. Are you taking pain medications sooner than the prescribed recommendations or taking more than the recommended amount at one time?

3. Are you unable to perform your usual daily activities because of either uncontrolled pain or effects of pain medication?

4. Do you find yourself going from one medical provider to another to get additional medications?

5. Are you lying to family members or health care providers in order to get additional medications?

6. Are you stealing money or medications from family or friends?

7. Are you using street drugs to supplement the prescribed medications?

8. Are you no longer able to perform daily activities or hold a job because of the pain or need for additional medications?

Once you determine there is a problem, start finding other methods of pain management and then get treatment for the addiction. Often times, there are solutions for chronic pain, such as surgery, exercise, holistic alternatives. Explore these options before engaging in long term use of narcotic pain killers. Keep in mind that there are many legitimate uses for narcotic pain medications. Cancer patients, especially once the cancer has moved into the bones, need to medicate sufficiently to relieve the pain. Many times elderly patients are limited in the choices they have to control pain. In these cases, addiction concerns are probably not at the forefront, but controlling the pain enough to promote at least a little more quality of life is the important consideration.

This discussion is not to totally discourage the use of narcotic pain medications, but to encourage the appropriate use of these powerful medications to control acute pain and promote healing. If you find that an acute pain condition becomes a chronic pain issue, advocate for yourself with your health care providers to insure that your pain treatments are going to be effective, and that you are able to maintain them over the long haul.

Surgeries
Over the course of this book, we have discussed some of the aspects to consider when faced with the choice of having surgery. In this section, we will discuss in more detail how to advocate for yourself in the world of surgical decisions and considerations. As stated earlier, there are three types of surgeries you can encounter; emergency surgery, elective surgery and non-elective surgery. Each type of surgery has its own considerations and will involve asking the right questions of your health care provider.

Let's start our discussion with emergency surgeries. These are surgeries that are generally undertaken in life threatening situations. In other words, if you do not have the surgery your life could and probably will be in danger. Some examples of emergency surgeries are: heart surgeries resulting from heart attacks, appendectomies, ruptured bowels, brain surgeries after a traumatic injury, broken bones where there is an open fracture or circulatory compromise, extreme skin or organ infections, ruptured aneurysms etc. Depending on the presenting condition and situation, you may not be the one making the decision to have the surgery. If you are unconscious, confused or for some reason unable to make an informed decision, a friend, spouse or family member may be asked to make the decision for you. If no one is present at the time and no one is reachable when a decision is needed, it is possible that the medical staff in charge of your care at the time may make the decision for you. If your life is hanging in the balance, this is going to be a good thing.

If you want to lower your risks of having a stranger make this decision for you, then there are a couple of things that you can do to be better prepared. Generally, even in most emergencies, patients either have their wallet and/or cell phone with them. Make sure that in your wallet you have a medical alert card that lists your medical history, medications, allergies and emergency contact phone numbers. Make sure that this information is up to date at all times. If you have a cell phone, and most people do these days, your cell phone has what is called an ICE number. ICE stands for In Case of Emergency. In this section of your phone, you can list the same information as on the medic alert card. Emergency personnel are trained to look for both of these items. Make sure that the people you have listed as your emergency contacts are aware of your medical history and wishes.

While some emergency surgeries are of an immediate nature, others will provide you with a little more time. Take this time to ask your health care provider about all of your options. It is best at this time to have a friend or family member in the room with you to verify what is actually being said. As a patient facing an emergency procedure, you may be experiencing some pretty significant anxiety and/or may be under the influence of medications that may cloud your perceptions and judgments. Another set of ears and eyes will come in handy in making a medically sound decision.

There are several questions that you should ask when faced with an emergency surgery:

1. What are the risks associated with the proposed surgery?

2. What are the risks of not having the proposed surgery?

3. How well equipped is the hospital to perform the type of surgery being proposed?

4. What are the surgeon's and hospital's infection rates and post-operative complication rates?

5. How long will you be staying in the hospital after the surgery?

6. How long is the typical recovery time from this type of surgery?

7. Is there time to get a second opinion?

8. Can you request a surgeon that you have a history with?

9. Does your surgeon have privileges at the hospital where you are?

10. Is there another hospital in town that is better equipped to do the surgery?

11. Is there time to be transferred to another facility if deemed appropriate?

12. Are there any risks associated with transferring to another facility?

13. Will your insurance cover transportation costs?

14. Does you insurance cover the procedure and has the hospital
    received pre-approval?

Asking these questions should help to raise your knowledge and
comfort level with the proposed surgery as well as minimize surprises.
Keep in mind, that in all but the most emergent circumstances, you
generally have some time and options. In many cities, there may be
several hospitals and each one usually has its specialties. Sometimes
a hospital will not provided the type of service you need and will tell
you they are going to transfer you to another facility. Most times you
will have a choice of where to go, but other times it will depend on the
availability of beds at the hospitals able to accommodate your needs.
While it is unfortunate that we must think about costs and insurance coverage, it is often better to think about this prior to making
the decisions listed above than be surprised when the bill comes and
nothing was covered. Most hospitals have the ability to predict with at
least some accuracy what procedures and facilities are covered by your
individual policy.

The second category of surgeries is the one called non-elective
surgeries. These surgeries if left unattended can lead to future problems or death. Many times, with non-emergent, non-elective surgeries,
you have a little more time to do your own research, get second opinions and select a facility and health care provider who you feel most
comfortable with. The questions you should be asking for non-elective
surgeries are very similar to the ones asked for emergent surgeries,
but here you have a few additional questions that you may want
answers to prior to agreeing to the surgery.

1. Are there any alternative procedures available? Remember earlier
   in the chapter we discussed making sure that your surgeon is
   capable of doing the most advanced and safest techniques available in your area. This decision can have a huge effect on your level
   of postoperative pain, recovery time, risk of complications and lost
   wages from longer recovery times.

2. What can you expect in terms of post-operative care after the
   surgery? Many times, there will be dressings you have to change.
   It is best to ask what materials you will need to have on hand after
   the surgery. You will also want to know when and how to change the
   dressings, and if this is something you will be able to do yourself or
   if you will need assistance. Even if you will require assistance from
   a family member, friend or home health care professional, you will
   want to know how things should be done so everyone is on the same
   page. Make sure that you get this information before the surgery,
   because you will have a better chance of retaining the information.
   If you wait until after the surgery, you will be tired, in pain and
   under the influence of medications that may affect your ability to
   learn and retain.

3. Will you need someone to stay with you and for how long? Knowing
   this beforehand will allow friends and family to plan time off work
   or to know when to schedule other family members or friends to
   help out.

4. When can you expect to be able to return to the various activities in
   your life? Make sure that you ask about any activity that is important to you such as showering, driving, returning to work, sports
   activities, sexual activities. Don't be afraid to have these frank
   discussions with your health care provider who is trained to answer
   these questions.

5. When should you follow up with your health care provider after
   surgery?

6. How frequently will you be required to follow up after the surgery?

7. What is the process for contacting your health care provider if there are problems or questions after the surgery?

8. What type of scars will be present after the surgery? What treatments are available to minimize the scarring?

9. What type of anesthesia will be used and/or are there options to pick from? Depending on the surgery, you may have choices in the type of anesthesia used. Some patients prefer to be completely oblivious to what is going on. Other patients prefer the least amount of anesthesia required.

10. How much post-operative pain can you expect?

11. How will the pain be treated in and out of the hospital?

12. What happens if the pain is not well controlled? What other actions can be taken to help reduce the pain?

The last type of surgery is the elective surgery. This is a surgery that you would like to have done to enhance some aspect of your health or appearance, but is not required to maintain health. Elective surgery is big business in this country. Many elective surgeries are generally safe, but keep in mind that all surgeries have risks. Before deciding to proceed with an elective surgery, make sure that you talk with the health care provider performing the surgery about all of the risks. Once you know the risks, ask yourself if you were to suffer one of the risks, would the surgery be worth it. The questions that you should ask of your health care provider prior to undertaking an elective surgery are the same for the emergent and non-elective surgeries.

Many of the elective surgeries performed in this country are for cosmetic purposes. While some people may think that undergoing elective cosmetic surgery for appearance enhancement is taking unnecessary risks with their overall health and well being, many people suffer both mentally and physically from certain cosmetic flaws. Take for example the patient who has lost a lot of weight and has a large amount skin that just hangs off his body. Not only does this affect the patient's self esteem, but it can put him at risk for painful and sometimes life threatening skin infections. Of course, this patient might consider the risks of the cosmetic surgery to eliminate the extra skin, less risky than suffering from the consequences of skin infections.

Many, if not most, of the risks associated with elective surgeries are the same as with any surgery or invasive procedure. Those risks include blood clots, infections, adverse anesthesia reactions, adverse post-operative drug reactions, improper or incomplete healing, scarring, disfigurement, and death. Depending on the procedure, some of the risks will be minimal, but always possible.

The best way to advocate for yourself for any type of surgery is to make sure that you question your health care provider thoroughly about the risks and how to minimize them. Question everyone involved in your care so that you are an informed consumer and to help insure that your health care provider is focusing on you. Make sure that you mark your own surgical spot when possible; to make sure that the correct area is being operated on. Every year despite increased safety measures being put in place by health care facilities, mistakes are still happening. These mistakes are not only the result of health care practitioners being careless, but patients being careless by not being diligent in making sure that their care providers are doing their jobs. Never leave anything to chance where your health care outcomes are concerned.

While there are many diseases that were not covered in this chapter and the diseases covered could have each been a book in themselves, it is hoped that you were able to garner a better look at how to handle whatever disease process you may encounter either personally or through a loved one. The main points, regardless of the disease, are to be involved in the management of your health care, be an active participant, don't be afraid to ask questions and have a trusted friend or family member available to help decipher the information. If you follow these simple steps, your ability to navigate the often complicated arena of health care management will be greatly enhanced.

Chapter 8

How to Survive a Stay in the Hospital

So you have done everything possible to avoid it, but you end up in the hospital anyway. In general, hospitals are wonderful places and the advancements in medical care have allowed us to live longer and healthier lives. With these advancements in health care, treatment procedures and surgical techniques, the length of hospital stays over the years has decreased greatly.

Let's start by looking at this subject from the patient's perspective. Many patients believe that hospital stays are being dictated by the insurance industry and that they, the patients, are being pushed out the door before they should be. There is some truth to this theory. Insurance companies realize that if patients leave the hospital sooner, their costs are going to be less. So, are the insurers just watching out for their bottom line or did they see trends in patient outcomes that indicated that longer hospital stays did not necessarily lead to better patient outcomes?

There is probably some truth on both sides of the argument. Certainly, if a patient spends less time in a hospital bed, the overall cost that the insurance companies are responsible for is going to be less. On the other hand, if the insurance industry saw that its costs were increasing because a majority of the patients had more complications after being discharged, they no doubt would approve longer stays. Part of what the insurance industry saw was that the longer patients remained in the hospital, the greater the chance that the patient was going to suffer some additional complications that would lead to even longer stays and higher costs. Health care providers also saw that the longer patients stayed in the hospital, the risk for additional complications increased. Those complications include increased risk of infection, skin breakdown, falls and accidents and unfortunately, medical care mistakes.

Contrary to popular belief, most health care providers prefer to see patients leave the hospital as soon as safely possible. This is because they have seen that patients often rest better in their home environment, are exposed to fewer infectious processes and are more motivated to participate in rehabilitation activities outside of the hospital confines. We will discuss more about some of these issues as we go through this chapter, but let's move on to some of the keys to surviving your hospital stay.

There are generally three ways that patients enter the hospital. The first way is through the emergency room. If you suffer a sudden onset of pain, illness or injury, you are likely to go through the emergency room for treatment and admission. The second way is through the surgery department. Generally, admission through the surgery department is on a non-emergency basis, and you have planned and discussed the procedure with your surgeon. The third way patients enter the hospital is through a direct admission on the advice of their primary medical care provider to manage an acute illness or to manage a chronic disease process that has flared up.

Regardless of how you enter the hospital, there are certain things that are essential to either have with you or available to insure that your wishes are followed and your medical treatment is appropriate and safe. Let's look at each of these things individually.

1. Advance directives – Regardless of age or health status, everyone
   should have at least a current, well thought out, Living Will and
   Durable Power of Attorney for Health Care. These documents help
   to insure that your wishes are followed. A Living Will is a declara-
   tion of what types of medical care or life saving or life preserving
   treatments you want. The Durable Power of Attorney for Health
   Care appoints a person or persons that you want to make medical
   decisions for you if you are unable or unwilling to make your own
   health care decisions.

   If you enter the hospital through the emergency room you may not
   have these documents on your person, but your emergency contact
   person should know where they are located and be able to bring a
   copy to the hospital as soon as possible. You should request that the
   hospital make a copy of these documents to be kept in your medical
   record. This process should be followed every time that you enter
   the hospital setting. You may be wondering why I recommend this
   should happen every time you enter the hospital if the hospital has
   a copy on file. There are several reasons. First, life changes, and you
   may have made changes to these documents since your last visit
   to the hospital. It is sometimes difficult to remember what copy is
   on file, and if the information is outdated by life changes such as
   divorce, death, etc. If the hospital has the wrong information on file
   and you are not in the condition to make these decisions, it is a good
   bet that your current wishes will not be followed.

   The second reason that you want to make sure that these documents are presented on every admission is because the hospital may
   not be able to find or retrieve the documents when needed. While
   most hospitals now have computerized medical records capabilities, it may not be possible to quickly retrieve the documents when
   needed. On occasion, wrong information is inputted into the system
   and your previous records will not be able to be accessed until the
   problem is corrected. Other times, medical personnel will not take
   the time to search previous records to find the documents, or they
   will find the documents but will not cross them over to your current
   medical record.

The third reason is that when you present these records to a member of the hospital team, she may make a copy and attach them to your current record but she doesn't make sure they are scanned and filed into the permanent medical record. You then operate under the assumption that your wishes are recorded in their system when in fact; they got lost in the process somewhere. When it comes to advance directives and your medical wishes, leave nothing to chance and make sure that you have these records available upon every admission to the hospital.

2. Medication Records – When entering the hospital, it is vitally important to have with you a list of your medications, the dosages and the number of times a day that you take them. This list should also include any over-the-counter medications, vitamins, nutritional supplements and herbal supplements. Once you have this information in hand, put it on a computer or computer disc so that it can be easily changed or regenerated when needed. Once you have printed the information, take it to an office supply store or printer to get it laminated to preserve it and keep it legible. This information then should be kept in your wallet and with you at all times. Make sure that any changes made to your medications or supplements are updated on your card at all times. This list should also include any drug, latex and food allergies that you have. If you have a cell phone, and most people do these days, this information can also be listed under the In Case of Emergency or ICE listing in your phone contacts. The advantages of listing this information in your cell phone are numerous. Most emergency personnel know to look in your phone for this information, it will generally always be with you and it is easy to update the information.

When making your list, pay particular attention to the spelling of the medications. Unfortunately, many medications have very similar spellings and a one letter difference can make a huge difference in the type of medication you receive while in the hospital. You will also want to pay attention to the dosage of the medication. Make sure that you know the difference between milligrams (mg) and micrograms (mcg). The abbreviations found on many medicine containers look very much alike. Milligrams are usually abbreviated to mg and micrograms are abbreviated mcg. When you are looking on the small print on the medicine bottles, it is often difficult to differentiate between the two. While there is only a one letter difference between the two abbreviations, the differences in the amount of medication is huge. The last thing that you want to pay attention to when doing your list is any decimal points that are part of your prescription. Once again these little dots are sometimes hard to see, but can make a huge difference in the amount of medication you receive.

So why is it so important to have this information with you when entering the hospital setting? Generally, regardless of how you enter the hospital, your stress levels are going to be high. When your stress levels are high, your memory tends to fail you. So, when the medical personnel asks you for your medications, you may not be able to remember the name, the spelling and/ or the dosage or you will give the wrong ones. This can lead to you receiving the wrong medications and/or dosages while in the hospital. Receiving the wrong medication or dosage will most definitely lead to complications, a longer hospital stay and, in the worst case scenario, life threatening consequences.

Let's take a look at the procedures that take place when you enter the hospital. The first step is, usually, a registered nurse will ask you for the list of your medications. The nurse will then write them in the chart. The doctor will review them and then order them during your stay. That list is then sent to the pharmacy and the medications are placed on the inpatient order sheet that the nurses on your admission unit will work from. You would think that with all of these checks and balances, nothing bad could possibly happen, but think again. If you start out giving the wrong information or, worse yet, no information, it will follow you through your entire hospitalization and perhaps even when you leave the hospital.

One client that I worked with entered the hospital through the emergency room. His wife gave the medication information to the nurse, but was not sure of the dose of her husband's antidepressant. Somehow instead of leaving the dosage blank, either the wife or the nurse assumed that the dosage was 20 milligrams per day. The patient was ordered the antidepressant at 20 milligrams per day. In reality, the dosage was to be 40 milligrams per day. This patient was sent home on the 20 milligram dose. This continued for six months before being caught. Unfortunately, this patient went six months being under medicated. Fortunately, for this patient, no harm was done, but imagine if the scenario was the other way around or the medication was for a problem of a more immediate life threatening nature.

Another example of what could go wrong in this process occurred when I was teaching student nurses in the clinical setting. Fortunately, for the patient, it was a nursing student who finally caught the problem before any harm was done. This patient too was brought in through the emergency room. He provided the ER nurse with his list of medications which included an herbal supplement that he took for prostate health. The dose of the medication was 1000mg four times per day. The nurse hand wrote this information on the ER notes. The resident who wrote inpatient orders could not read the nurse's handwriting and instead of verifying the information with the patient, ordered a blood pressure medication at 1000 mgs four times a day. The typical dose of the blood pressure medication ordered, was 50 mgs per day. Keep in mind, this patient did not have a recorded history of high blood pressure. So, not only did this patient get ordered a medication that he did not take or need, but it was ordered at 80 times the normal dosage. This mistake made it through the pharmacy checkpoint without being caught. The medication was placed into the patient's medication box. Fortunately, the nursing student was aware of the appropriate dosage and asked the patient if that was the dose he normally took. The patient stated that he did not have high blood pressure and never took that medication. In this case, had the student nurse not been diligent in telling the patient what kind of medication she was giving him and questioning him about the dose, this patient could have very easily died from this mistake.

These examples illustrate the importance of making sure that you are prepared when you enter the hospital system. Even though hospitals are implementing more and more checks and balances to prevent these kinds of mistakes, you can see that even with four levels of checks and balances, mistakes are still happening. These mistakes are not just rare exceptions, but are happening everyday in just about every hospital in the country. Your safety starts and ends with you. Do not leave anything to chance. Once you have given your medications to the hospital personnel, ask to see the list, and once the doctor has written the orders, make sure that you ask to look at the medications ordered and verify that your regular medications are correct. Also, don't be afraid to ask about any additional medications ordered. These simple steps will help to protect you against medication errors and unwanted health complications.

3. A Patient Advocate – The third thing that you want to have with you when you enter the hospital is someone to advocate for you and with you. This can be a family member, friend or professional patient advocate. This person or persons should be with you as much as possible to be an extra set of ears, take notes and pay attention to what is going on when you are unable to. You can, when able, advocate for yourself by being an active participant in your health care. Make sure that you are asking questions throughout your entire hospital stay. Always ask what medications you are getting and how much. Ask about the tests you are receiving and what to expect during the testing. If there is something that you don't understand or can't spell or pronounce, have the medical provider write it down for you. Keep a notebook handy so that you and/or your advocate can keep track of everything.

So we now know what the three things are that you must have anytime you enter the hospital. Now let's look at some of the other things you can do that will help you survive your hospital stay.

Read and Understand Before You Sign

When you enter the hospital system, you will be asked to sign a number of papers. Some of these papers are informational and some are legally binding, so make sure you know what you are signing to avoid surprises down the road. Let's take a look at some of the papers that you may be asked to sign.

Consent to treat forms
These forms state that you are giving the health care facility permission to treat you. Read this form carefully to know exactly what you are giving permission for. You may be asked to sign more than one of these forms and generally they will be slightly different and may cover very specific procedures. An example would be an additional consent form for a test, procedure or surgery. These forms should specifically spell out the risks and benefits of the treatment. Make sure that you read the entire form and understand what risks you may face. If you do not understand some of the words or concepts, make sure to ask for an explanation before signing.

Privacy forms
These forms will explain your privacy rights and how and to whom your medical information may be shared. Once again, it is important to understand this information and read the forms in their entirety. Most of the privacy forms will be very similar in nature and are basically an insurance policy for the health care facility to show that they have disclosed to you how the information is shared and protected.

Release of information forms

When signing these forms, you are designating who may access your medical records for continuity of care, record keeping, legal purposes, etc. An example of how this form may be used is if you were to go to one hospital after being seen at another hospital. The hospital that you are currently in will request information from the hospital where you were previously seen. This will help them to avoid duplicating tests and give them a better background of your medical history. These forms may also contain the names of friends or family members that you designate to be kept informed about your medical care.

Financial responsibility forms

These forms are generally signed when you enter the health care facility to state that you are responsible for paying the bill. The forms explain your rights in determining if your bill is correct, what happens if your insurance company refuses to pay, payment options and actions that the health care facility can take against you if you fail to pay for services rendered. Read these forms thoroughly and understand what you are signing before signing it.

If you are concerned about being able to afford your care, ask for information on financial services that the health care facility has available.

Patient rights forms

Many hospitals will provide you with a copy of the patient bill of rights and will ask you to sign this form to prove they have informed you of your rights and responsibilities as a patient. This is always useful information to have so that you know what to expect and your responsibilities as a patient.

Personal Belongings Form

This form lists the items that you came to the hospital with. Look over this form carefully to make sure that all of your belongings are listed. When leaving the hospital, check over the list again and make sure that you are leaving with everything you came with. We will discuss a little more about personal belongings in the hospital later in this chapter.

Discharge Instruction Forms

These forms will explain the information you will need to know once you leave the hospital. Read these forms from top to bottom to make sure that you know what to expect after leaving the hospital. Prior to signing this form, make sure that you ask the discharge staff to explain anything you don't understand.

Reduce Your Risk of Infection

Hospitals generally pride themselves on cleanliness, but don't be fooled by appearances. Hospitals are breeding grounds for many infectious processes. While you cannot control all of your exposures to infections, there are a few things that you can do to minimize your risk by following the steps listed below.

Examine your environment

When you first enter the hospital, look around at the environment of the hospital. Does it appear clean? Does it smell clean? Are there people cleaning? Is there trash in the trash cans? Are there dirty linens lying around? Do the linens on your bed look and smell clean? Are the floors clean? Are the bed rails and bed frames clean? Are the bathrooms clean? Do you see spots or stains on the floors, walls, curtains and/or furniture? Is there used equipment in the room? Are the monitors that are used in your care clean?

Looking for the above mentioned items will help guide you in determining whether the hospital truly values its cleanliness. In some cases, you may look around and decide to walk out and try another hospital. Often this won't be a choice because of the circumstances that brought you to the hospital in the first place. If you find yourself in the hospital and you see something that you don't feel has been cleaned, then by all means ask the staff to either clean the area appropriately or ask to be moved to another room.

The one area of the hospital that often poses the greatest risk of infection is the emergency room. One reason is that when people come to the ER they are sick and many have some sort of infection whether it is a cold, flu, strep throat, pneumonia, stomach infection, skin infection or bug infestation. You name the infection and every ER in the country has probably seen it at one point or another during the day. Another reason ER's are breading grounds for infection is they are generally busy places with fast turnovers, and in the process of turning rooms over fast, things don't always get cleaned the way they should. By all means, if you enter an ER and things don't look clean, tell someone about it.

Make sure that your health care providers are washing their hands

Everyone that comes into your room should be washing his hands before touching you and/or anything in your environment. Do not be afraid to remind your health care providers about this if you do not physically witness them cleaning their hands. If you are in a semi-private room with another patient, make sure that your health care providers are cleaning their hands in between contacts with the other patient and you. Also, make sure that your health care providers are washing their hands when they go from performing one task on you to performing another task where their hands or gloves are coming into contact with bodily fluids.

Many hospitals have now implemented the alcohol based hand washes in just about all rooms and public areas. This is a very effective way of hand cleaning and one that I feel is, in most cases, preferable over the soap and water method. With the soap and water method, many health care providers do not wash their hands long enough to truly be effective. They squirt some soap on the hands, run it under water for a few seconds and they are done. When hand washing is done in this manner, it is usually not an effective method of infection control. The alcohol based hand gels are quicker, more effective and usually come with a higher level of compliance than the soap and water method. If your health care provider should have blood, body fluids or other visible soil on their hands, then they should use soap and water for a minimum of 30 seconds.

Make sure that friends and family members do the same
If your friends or family members come to visit you, make sure that they, too, are using either the alcohol based hand wash or soap and water every time they enter or leave the room. The last thing you want is your friends or family making your condition worse by bringing unnecessary germs into your environment.

Don't forget your own hands
You, too, should be sure that you are keeping your hands as clean as possible to avoid spreading germs to yourself or others that enter your room. If you are unable to get out of bed to use the sink or hand cleaning dispensers, then ask a friend or family member to bring you in a personal container of hand cleaner. You can also ask the hospital personnel to bring you a basin with soap and water to keep up with the task.

Make sure that the tools are clean
Stethoscopes are one of the most common tools used by doctors and nurses and unfortunately, a tool that does not get cleaned often enough. Don't be afraid to ask your health care provider to wipe down their stethoscope or other assessment tools before using them on you.

Go private when possible
If you have a choice between a hospital with all private rooms or one that has semi-private rooms, all else being equal, go for the one with the private rooms. Whether it is a hospital or extended care facility, being in a room by yourself helps to cut down on infection. One reason is you will not be exposed to any infectious

processes that a roommate or the roommate's visitors may bring with them. Secondly, there is less chance of cross contamination from your health care providers and another patient. If you must share a room with someone, make sure that your roommate does not have a contagious infection. If you suspect that your roommate has something that you don't, or something you don't want to get, request to be transferred to another room.

Beware of the urinary catheter

Many times in hospitals, patients are provided with urinary catheters due to an inability to urinate, immobility, recovery from a surgical procedure and/or fluid balance monitoring. Two reasons not to have a catheter are for staff convenience and/or patient convenience. Urinary catheters are one of the leading causes of hospital acquired infections and these infections are mostly preventable with proper use and care. Fortunately, more health care providers are using greater discretion in the use of urinary catheters, but there are others who are still ordering them unnecessarily and people who are not using the appropriate technique to insert them.

If your health care provider orders a catheter for you, don't be afraid to ask if it is absolutely necessary. If it is necessary for your care, then make sure that the person inserting the catheter is using the proper technique. The procedure should always be done using a sterile technique. If the health care provider does not get it in on the first attempt, make sure she is getting a new catheter and not using the same one twice. Your health care provider may tell you that she has cleaned it off, but this is still not acceptable and greatly increases your risk of infection. Once the catheter is in, it is important to make sure that it is getting cleaned on a regular basis. Catheter care should be done at least twice a day using soap and water. The area should be cleaned from front to back to avoid cross contamination. If you do not feel comfortable with the health care provider performing this task, you can request that they teach you how to do this yourself. If you chose and are able to perform this task for yourself, make sure that you do it at least twice a day using the appropriate technique.

The last word of advice is to make sure that the catheter is taken out as soon as medically safe. Leaving a catheter in for too long greatly increases the risk of infection. Keep in mind, keeping a catheter in because it is easier for the patient or staff, is not an acceptable method of health care practice.

Beware of the IV catheter
Another type of catheter that is often used in hospitals is the IV catheter. These catheters can also be a great source of infection and other untoward complications. The scary thing about infections caused by IV catheters is they often can enter the blood stream. Once an infectious agent has entered the blood stream, the complications can come fast and furiously and are often difficult to treat successfully. There are several different types of intravenous catheters from the peripheral IV that is left in up to three days to surgically implanted catheters that can be used for more long term therapies for the chronically ill patient.

Make sure that, once again, you ask your health care provider if an IV is absolutely necessary. Once necessity is established, then make sure that the person or persons inserting the device are doing so properly. The site where the catheter is to be placed should be cleaned thoroughly and if the medical provider is not successful on the first attempt, then new equipment should be used for subsequent tries.

Once the IV is in place, the health care providers should be assessing the site on a frequent basis to check for signs of infection and/or other complications. If you notice any pain, redness or swelling at the site, make sure that you notify someone immediately to have the catheter removed. Every time that medication is given through the catheter the site should be cleaned and flushed. If this does not happen, bring it to the attention of your health care provider. Overall, IV therapy is a safe and effective tool in health care management, but care and diligence should always be practiced to avoid unwarranted complications.

Keep your lungs free of infection

Pneumonia is another huge source of hospital acquired infections. There are several ways to get pneumonia while in the hospital. The first way is to be cross contaminated by other patients who have the disease either by direct contact with these patients or by your health care providers carrying the bacteria into your room. This is why it is important to make sure that everyone entering your room practices good hand hygiene, and that they wipe down all equipment, such as stethoscopes, blood pressure cuffs and oxygen monitors, before using them on you.

The second way to get pneumonia is from lying in a hospital bed for extended periods of time. When you are in the hospital because of injury, disease and/or pain, you tend to spend the bulk of your time in bed on your back. When this happens, the secretions that are normally generated by the lungs, start to pool in the base of the lungs and the longer they pool there, the greater the chance of bacterial growth that can lead to pneumonia. Pain is also a precursor to pneumonia because when you are in severe pain, you are guarded and do not take the deep breaths necessary to keep the lungs properly inflated. If you are receiving medication to help with the pain, you may be able to breathe more easily but will probably not breathe as deeply because the pain medication is stunting your breathing effort.

To avoid this type of pneumonia, try to move around as much as possible even if it is getting up and sitting in a chair for a while. If you are able to walk around, that, too, will help stimulate breathing and keep those secretions at bay. The other way to prevent pneumonia is to be compliant with the breathing exercises that are provided in the hospital. Most hospitals will provide all their patients with a device called an Incentive Spirometer. An Incentive Spirometer is a tube-like device that encourages a patient to inhale deeply to move a marker in the tube. Make sure that you are provided with this tool whenever you are in the hospital or bedridden for a prolonged period of time.

Don't be a victim of bed sores

Another source of infection that is unfortunately acquired in hospital and nursing facilities are bed sores, also referred to as pressure ulcers. The sad thing is these are totally preventable. With proper turning, hydration and skin care, bed sores and the resulting skin and systemic infections caused by them can be prevented. If you or a loved one is bedridden for any length of time, make sure that turning is occurring at least every two hours, skin is kept dry and the body properly hydrated.

Whether we like it or not, hospitals can be breeding grounds for infections, and while the above suggestions may not prevent all hospital acquired infections, they should cut your risks greatly. As with anything regarding your health care, you have to become an active participant and ask questions and speak up when necessary.

Make Sure You Are Getting the Right Medications

Medication errors have been the bane of the health care field for years. Hospitals, pharmacies and health care providers are constantly trying to come up with ways to prevent these mistakes, but yet, they keep happening. Health care providers are increasing their use of electronically generated prescriptions to cut down on handwriting errors. Hospitals and pharmacies are relying more heavily on computer technology to help with more reliable checks and balances. If you have been in a hospital lately, you probably noticed that your health care providers are scanning both medications and patients to insure more accurate administration of medications. You may ask yourself, why, with all of the technology and checks and balances, are the mistakes continuing? Even with technology, it comes down to human error. If the wrong data is put into the computers, the wrong data will come out of the computers.

So how can you as a patient or health advocate for a loved one make sure that these mistakes don't happen to you? The main way is to be an active participant in your health care or have an advocate participate when you are unable. I cannot tell you how many patients come into the health care system with a list of medications and have no idea why they are taking the medications. Below are some things you can do when advocating for yourself or a loved one when it comes to medications.

1. When entering the hospital have that list of medications that we discussed earlier. Look at your list and make sure that you know why you are taking each medication.

2. When someone comes into your room with a handful of medications, ask what each medication is, what it is for and what the dose is. If any of the answers don't sound right, ask more questions. If someone tells you one of the medications is for high blood pressure and you have no history of high blood pressure, ask why you are receiving that medication. If you do not get a sufficient answer, refuse to take the medication until it has been clarified. This is particularly important when sharing a hospital room with another patient. Make sure that the health care provider has the right patient.

3. Take only medications that you need. As we discussed earlier, every medication has side effects that may require additional medications. When it comes to medications, less is often better. Do not be afraid to question your health care providers about the necessity of medications. Remember, that many health care providers profit from the number of diagnoses and prescriptions that they can come up with. If you are in the hospital and the health care provider wants to give a pain medication and you are experiencing no pain, refuse the medication. On the other hand, if you are in pain, take the medication to keep the pain from getting out of control. If the

health care provider wakes you up to give you something to help you sleep, think twice.

4. Make sure that you know the names of the medications that you are allergic to. Know both the generic and trade names of your allergies. Many health care providers will use the generic name when referring to medications so it is important that you know both. If you are allergic to a certain ingredient in a medication, make sure that you are aware of other drugs that contain that same ingredient to insure that you are not exposed to the allergen. Make sure that the health care facility provides you with an allergy bracelet and that the staff is checking it before administering the medications.

5. Be an active participant in your health care. Ask questions, question your health care providers and know what you are getting and why. Remember, you have the right to refuse medications until you receive the clarifications that you request. Do not be bullied into taking something that you do not believe to be the right medication for you.

Don't Lose a Good Body Part

We have all heard or read about patients who have gone to the hospital and had the wrong body part operated on or removed. Having the wrong part operated on is usually a correctable error, but having the wrong body part removed is indeed a tragic event. It seems impossible that these kinds of mistakes happen, but they do. These events happen when someone marks x-rays or other diagnostic tests with the wrong side. The other problem occurs when surgeons flip these pictures the wrong way. This problem can also occur when the wrong records get sent in with the patient. Once again, health care facilities have taken many steps to avoid these harrowing mistakes. Many facilities have instituted a process called a "time out", where the health care providers stop and perform a series of checks and balances. These same facilities are requesting that the patient mark the operative spot when possible. Below is a list of things that you can do to make sure that you are not a victim of one of these tragedies.

1. Be involved in your care. Take the time to make sure the right body part is getting marked or you are marking it yourself. Make sure that you know which part it is. I know this sounds a little ridiculous, but some patients really don't know when they get to the hospital. This happens a lot with internal organs where the patient may not be experiencing pain or other symptoms, but something has been found during diagnostic testing. When discussing the surgery with your health care provider, make sure that you familiarize yourself with the planned procedure and don't be afraid to repeatedly question the medical provider on the location.

2. Make sure the medical records the health care providers are working from are yours. If necessary, ask to see the chart and make sure that it contains your name, and that the identifying information is correct.

3. When possible, make sure that you talk to your surgeon immediately prior to your surgery time to make sure that you both are still on the same page. You should also be talking to the anesthesiologist prior to the procedure. This person will be yet another part of the checks and balances.

4. Make sure you know who is going to be operating on you. You may think it is the surgeon that you have been dealing with, but many hospitals have residents or students that work with the surgeons. While everyone has to learn sometime, be sure if there is going to be a resident in the room, you know what her role is going to be. If you feel uncomfortable about a resident conducting the bulk of your surgery, request that the surgeon performs the surgery. Remember, you are the boss and have the right to know and chose who will be performing your procedures.

5. Prior to going into surgery, make sure that you have a name band on, and everyone involved with your care is checking the information on that band. If you have medication or material allergies, make sure that you have an allergy band on and they are checking that as well.

Following these simple steps will help you avoid a devastating medical error.

Getting the Rest You Need and Deserve

You have either experienced firsthand or heard the horror stories of how difficult it is to get rest in the hospital due to nurses, doctors, nursing students, medical students, blood draws, testing, vital signs, meals, housekeepers, nurse's aides, visitors and generally lots of noise. With all of these distractions going on 24 hours a day, rest is difficult. While you don't want to be disturbed every time you get to sleep, you also want to receive the appropriate care while in the hospital. Once again, remember you are the customer and the boss. Following the steps below will help to increase the rest you receive during your hospital stay.

1. Request that hospital staff coordinate their care as much as possible to avoid distractions. Many times the health care providers can take care of their assessments, medications and procedures at one time.

2. Ask that care is coordinated with meal times so that you can sleep in between.

3. When feeling tired and wanting to sleep, ask that a do not disturb sign be put on your door.

4. Feel free to be honest with visitors. If you are tired and do not feel like visiting, ask that your visitors leave or have the staff put a sign on the door requesting visitors to check with the nurse before entering your room.

5. If you have a friend or family member that is staying with you or advocating for you, make sure that you tell them when you need rest and require quiet, or have them leave the room for a while. They, too, will probably appreciate a break now and then.

6. Request that your door stay shut to cut down on hospital noises. If keeping the door shut is not possible, request a pair of ear plugs to cut down on the ambient noises.

7. Get out as soon as safely possible. Getting out of the hospital is generally going to be the best way to get rest. Of course, if you are a parent of small children and/or have a spouse or significant other who is not particularly helpful, a hospital stay may seem like a vacation.

8. Take a favorite pillow or blanket with you that may be more comfortable than those provided by the hospital.

Getting the Care that You Need and Deserve

Getting quality health care while in a hospital should be an expectation not an exception. The higher the quality of your day to day care, the happier you will be and the more quickly you will recover. As a patient and customer, you should take several steps to insure top notch care.

1. When possible, check out the hospital before checking in. If you have a preplanned hospital visit coming up, talk with friends, family and health care providers to get their opinions on which hospitals provide the best services. There are also many web sites in most cities that rank hospitals in many care areas such as hospital acquired infections, falls, medical errors, safety violations/compliances, nurse-to-patient ratios and/or cleanliness/health violations.

2. Once in the hospital, be involved and proactive in your care. Ask questions and know what is going on and/or have someone do this for you if you are not able.

3. Treat the staff with respect, and request that they, too, treat you with respect and honor your wishes and privacy.

4. Be compliant with appropriate medical recommendations and treatments. You are there for a reason, and for the most part, the treatments ordered by your health care providers are for your care and safety. If the health care provider has requested that you not eat or drink anything, then don't have friends and family sneaking in contraband.

5. Make sure that the staff is getting you up and moving when appropriate to avoid blood clots, infections, constipation and bed sores.

6. When physically unable to move around by yourself, make sure that you request staff assistance when moving around your room.

7. Make sure that the staff provide you with a call light to summon help or assistance when needed. If you feel that the staff is not answering call lights in a timely fashion, ask to speak with your nurse. If the nurse is the source of the problem and does not have a good explanation, ask to talk with the nursing supervisor. Sometimes the nurse will be busy with other patients and a member of the ancillary staff will answer the call light. If you wish to speak with the nurse, when possible, tell the ancillary staff what it is you want. This will save the nurse time and help to ensure your requests get addressed as soon as possible.

8. Make sure that you are getting the proper nutrition while hospitalized. A major part of the healing process is getting the nutrients the body needs to heal. If your food is cold or not edible for some reason, ask for a new tray or for your tray to be reheated. If your health care provider has requested that you eat a special diet, then make sure that any foods that family or friends bring in meet the

diet criteria. If you are in the hospital for problems with your gall bladder and your family brings you a double-bacon cheeseburger, be prepared to pay the price.

9. When getting discharged, pay close attention to the discharge instructions so that you are comfortable in continuing your care at home. Insist that the staff involved in your discharge sits down and takes the appropriate time to explain things and answer questions. If you are to be sent home with dressings, drains, catheters and/ or IVs, make sure that you know what you should be doing. Make sure that the staff asks you to repeat the information or do a return demonstration of treatment explanations. Things seem really simple when you are in the hospital and someone else is doing it, but it is a whole different story once you get home and try doing it for yourself.

10. Before being discharged, make sure that you have and understand any and all arrangements for home health care if it is needed. It is much easier to get things worked out when you have the resources in front of you than trying to figure it out for yourself at home. If you feel that you need additional services and they have not been offered, request to speak with a social worker/discharge planner.

11. If you are to be discharged to a skilled nursing facility for additional care and rehabilitation and know this in advance, do your homework on the reputable nursing homes in your area. If you are unable to do this beforehand, then ask a friend or family member to research the facilities for you. Nursing homes, unfortunately, are not created equal. There is nothing worse than to survive a visit to the hospital just to be done in by a poorly skilled nursing facility. You can ask the hospital staff to recommend a place, but keep in mind their goal is to get you out and turn over the bed, so chances are they will recommend the place that affords them the quickest and easiest discharge. We will discuss how to pick the right nursing home in a latter chapter.

12. If you have financial questions or problems paying for the care you received while in the hospital, ask to speak to a financial counselor before leaving the hospital. Most hospitals will have financial assistance programs available to help defer some of the costs. They can also work with your insurance company to make sure that as much as possible gets paid. Once out of the hospital, remember you can always call and talk to the billing department and negotiate lower rates. Many cities now have web sites that will list the costs of certain services in your area and provide you with more ammunition for negotiating charges.

13. Remember to get out of the hospital as soon as safely possible. The longer you stay, the more you are at risk for complications.

Leave With What You Came With

Leave with what you came with. Patient belongings are forever getting lost in hospitals. To keep your valuables safe, leave them home whenever possible. When you do have to take something to the hospital with you, make sure that your name and phone number is written on the item. Let's look at some of the items that are commonly lost in the hospital.

1. Jewelry- Jewelry should be left at home or sent home with a trusted friend or family member. Many people don't like to part with wedding rings or religious medals while in the hospital, but the fact is, there is a good chance they will get lost. For many tests and surgeries, jewelry must be removed for patient safety and testing accuracy. When these items are removed, they will get placed in a bag or container and put somewhere. Chances are you may not be in the frame of mind to remember to ask for them back, and the staff will likely forget about them, as well. The other problem is patients may experience weight gain or loss while in the hospital which affects the fit of the jewelry. Weight gain and swelling while wearing jewelry can result in compromised circulation leading to physical complications and requiring the jewelry be cut to prevent

additional injury. If weight loss is experienced, jewelry may become loose and get lost in the linens.

2. Medications – Many patients like to bring their medications with them to the hospital. It is generally best to just bring a list of the medications. Once again, medications can get lost and in some cases stolen. There is nothing worse than just having your prescriptions refilled and then have the medications disappear. Often, patients believe that it will be cheaper if they take their own medications while in the hospital. While there may be some truth to this, you greatly increase your risk of medication errors. So you may save yourself some money on the medication administration, but end up with a bigger bill related to complications from the higher risks of medication errors, duplications/overdoses and theft.

3. Electronics/phones – It is nice to have something to keep you distracted while lying around in a hospital bed, but unfortunately these are often very desirable items for people to take. Keep in mind that you will be under the influence of medications that will make you sleepy. You will also be out of the room for tests and procedures giving any number of people an opportunity to walk off with your favorite diversions. If you must have a phone or other electronic device with you, leave it with a friend or family member when you are out of the room or cover it up and leave it in a drawer. Make sure that when you return to your room that all of your belongings are where you left them.

4. Dentures, Glasses, Hearing Aids and Prosthetics – These are usually items that people do not like to be without. You need your glasses to read information related to your care. Dentures help you to eat and get the proper nutrition. Hearing aids are vital for hearing what is going on around you and being able to hear and understand instructions and information that you are given. Prosthetics may be needed for walking, eating, etc. So, these are some of the items that you will want to keep with you in the hospital and are generally items that are personally adapted enough not be used or desired by others. While these items may not be ripe for stealing, they often get lost in trash cans and linens.

Make sure that when you are not using these items that they are placed in a drawer where they cannot be knocked off into the trash or sent to the laundry in the linens.

5. Money – Generally, you do not need much money while in the hospital. If you want to keep a few dollars with you to buy a newspaper or something at the gift shop, keep it in a drawer and keep it to a minimum. If you should enter the hospital in an emergency situation or don't have anyone to send your money and credit cards home with, then ask to keep these items in the hospital safe.

6. Clothing – Clothing is another thing that can be kept to a minimum. The hospital will provide you with your own personal designer gown. These gowns make it easier for the health care providers to get to the areas that they need to get to. If you want to wear something more comfortable and less revealing, make it something loose fitting and nothing of great value. Many times in the hospital there will be bleeding, drainage and various other bodily fluids and substances that may ruin your favorite lounge wear. If you come into the hospital in an emergency situation, you may find that your favorite outfit has ended up in the trash. In this case, thank your lucky stars that the staff thought more of you than your clothes.

7. Changing rooms- Often in the hospital you will be transferred between different areas or rooms. Make sure that every time you are moved, a friend, family member or staff member gathers all of your belongings and checks them against the belongings list that you filled out upon admission. If something comes up missing, report it to a staff member and have them check your previous room or the lost and found area.

8. Making a claim – If you should lose something while in the hospital, you can file a report with the facility's risk management department. If you can prove that the item was stolen or lost by a staff member, you may get some sort of reimbursement. Hospitals, of course, try to keep their number of claims down and this is why they encourage you not to keep too many valuables with you.

Chapter 9

Advance Directives, Legal and Financial Health Planning

Throughout the book, the term advance directives has been mentioned several times as well as the importance of having these documents in place to better insure that your health care wishes are carried out. In addition, it is important to consider various other legal and financial issues that may impact your general health, mental health, family health and financial health. You may be asking why advanced legal and financial planning is being addressed in a book about personal health advocacy. Unfortunately or fortunately, depending on how you look at it, our legal and financial health often can dictate our physical and mental health, as can our physical and mental health have a huge impact on our legal and financial health.

This chapter will address the different advance directives in a general overview. We will also look at some of the things that you can do to better protect yourself and your finances related to health care, insurance and planning for the various stages of life. While this chapter will not go into specific legal and financial planning, we will provide an overview and recommendations on where to turn to get the advice necessary to navigate the often complex options that most of us will be faced with at some point in the life span. Keep in mind as you go through this chapter that the information here is a general overview and laws and services vary from state to state. We recommend that you become familiar with the specifics of the state you or your loved ones live in.

Advance Medical Directives

If we look at the anatomy of the term advanced medical directives, what it is saying is that we are setting forth a set of directives that we want executed at some point in the future. We are setting these directives in advance in case, at some point, we are unable to direct our own care but desire that our wishes are followed in a way which we feel is appropriate for our individual needs.

It is never too early to start planning for the future. An eighteen year old individual is generally not going to be thinking about the "what ifs" in life, but unfortunately we never know what the future has in store for us. At this age, generally parents are still going to be making the calls if the unthinkable happens, but some in this age group have already developed specific thoughts related to their health care. If you are of legal age, then you need to start thinking about your desires related to health care, and get them in writing with the legal documents recognized by the health care industry in your state.

Living Wills
The first legal document related to health care that we will look at is the Living Will. The Living Will can be general in nature or you can make it as specific as you want. Most health care facilities such as hospitals, assisted living facilities and nursing homes will provide you with materials that explain your choices where living wills are concerned. The Living Will documents that you can fill out in most health care facilities, will suit most people's needs, but it is also something that you should read over carefully to make sure that you understand what you are signing.

A Living Will addresses your wishes if you are deemed to be in a state of health where death is imminent. There are several choices that

you can make as part of your Living Will. The one choice that you
can make is that you want all possible life sustaining and life saving
actions taken regardless of your diagnosis. That means, that even if
you are in a permanent vegetative state or have a life ending illness,
that you want to be kept alive as long as possible. The other choice
states that you do not want life sustaining or life saving measures
taken if your doctor and another doctor deem that your condition is
terminal. These measures usually involve feeding tubes, artificial
respiration, etc. You, of course, can also choose any combination of life
sustaining activities. In some states, Living Wills will ask you if you
wish to be an organ donor. It helps to have this designation in writing
if it is your wish so that your family members and loved ones don't
have to make that decision during an already stressful time.

When reading over your options in a Living Will, it is important to
understand when the Living Will will be enforced. Let's look at an
example where confusion often occurs. In your Living Will, you have
stated that you do not want a feeding tube to provide nutrition to
prolong your life. If your condition is not considered to be terminal, but
instead temporary, you may very well desire to have a feeding tube. An
example would be in the case of a stroke where your ability to swallow
effectively is hampered by the stroke. The ability to swallow may
return in time with therapy and treatment, and the feeding tube will
provide you with the nutrition necessary to heal and regain some of
those abilities. Artificial respiration is often another area of confusion.
Many patients believe that once they are placed on a ventilator, they
will never come off. In many cases this is not true. There are many
times when a ventilator is used only to stabilize a condition and then
is discontinued.

The main thing to understand about Living Wills is that they are
activated during the end of life. It would be impossible for you to write
every possible provision into a Living Will, but if there are certain
things that you feel strongly about, make sure that you legally modify
the Living Will document for your state to address those issues.
Once you have completed your Living Will and have it witnessed or
notarized, depending on the state you live in, make copies. One copy

should be kept in your files and be clearly marked so that someone can easily locate the document. You should also provide copies to your loved ones who are likely to be around when a health crisis strikes. You will also want to take a copy with you anytime you enter any kind of health care facility (hospital, surgery center, emergency room, rehab facility, retirement community, assisted living facility and/or nursing home). Another place to keep a copy is in a Vial of Life packet or emergency medical file. Once you have completed your Living Will, you should make sure that you review it on a regular basis to make sure that it still reflects your wishes. As you age, as your health changes, or as there are changes in your living situation, you may want to make changes to reflect your current wishes.

Durable Power of Attorney for Health Care

As stated above, a Living Will deals with your wishes at the end of life, but it does not cover you if you are unable or unwilling to make your own health care decisions during times of accident or illness. When this happens, it helps to have a Durable Power of Attorney for Health Care. This document appoints someone of your choice to make those decisions for you.

When appointing a Durable Power of Attorney for Health Care, it should be someone who you trust to make health care decisions for you and someone you have talked with regarding your wishes. If you explain your wishes and the person that you want to appoint disagrees or expresses problems with carrying out your wishes, then it would be better to come up with someone else. This appointee should be familiar and in agreement with the wishes expressed in your Living Will. Your Durable Power of Attorney for Health Care can override your Living Will if she so chooses.

Make sure that you are familiar with the laws regarding Durable Power of Attorney for Health Care rules in your state. Some states and some medical facilities will honor these agreements differently. In most states, a patient does not have to be declared legally incompetent for the document to take effect. This document can take effect when a person decides that he no longer feels comfortable making his own health care decisions. It can also take effect in the case of accident or illness that prohibits the patient from speaking on his own behalf. It can also be enacted when the patient is under the influence of mind altering medications, mental illness, dementia, Alzheimer's, alcoholism or any other condition that prohibits the person from understanding treatment options and/or making sound health care decisions for himself.

When making a choice in appointing your Durable Power of Attorney for Health Care, it is important to appoint someone who is knowledgeable about your health history and health care needs and has the time to devote to making sure that you are getting the appropriate health care. This person should be available when needed and should also be willing to go toe to toe with health care providers to insure that your care is appropriate and needed. Unfortunately, when people enter the health care system without someone to advocate for them, chances are the overall care that they receive will be subpar.

If someone you know or love has asked you to be her Durable Power of Attorney for Health Care, you should take the responsibility seriously. If you do not feel comfortable with this level of responsibility, don't have the time to devote to the job should it become necessary or don't feel that you can understand and make the appropriate decisions, it is important to speak up before it is too late. If you do decide to take on the responsibility, make sure that you have had the appropriate discussions with the person doing the appointing. If you should have to act on someone's behalf, then make sure that you get as many facts as possible before making decisions. Be active in monitoring the person's health care and make sure that you develop positive relationships with the person's health care providers.

There are several problems that you can run into with the Durable Power of Attorney for Health Care. There are times when the health care providers don't honor the designee's wishes where the patient's care is concerned. There are some health care providers who don't believe that the designation kicks in until the patient is declared incompetent. Many doctors believe that they are the ultimate decision makers in the patient's care and have final authority in decisions. Since health care is not an exact science and many things are left to interpretation, these issues are at times difficult to resolve. Let's look at several examples of issues that arise when the Durable Power of Attorney for Health Care comes into question.

I, myself, had problems when my mother entered a nursing home for physical therapy for knee pain. When a patient enters an extended care facility, the admission orders are generally written by the patient's primary care physician or the hospital's discharging physician. Once the patient is admitted to the extended care facility, that facility's doctor will review the orders and usually change them as he sees fit. In my mother's case, her primary care physician had written the orders and had sought my guidance in her care. When I delivered my mother to the facility, I informed them that I wanted those orders to be followed and that I wanted to be consulted prior to any changes to the orders. The day after admission, my mother called me very confused and agitated. I wondered what had happened.

When I arrived at the facility to see what was going on, I stopped at the nurse's station to inquire if there had been any changes to her orders. The nurse informed me that the facility's physician had ordered a new pain medication and an anti-depressant. When I inquired why, the nurse stated that the doctor had spent a few minutes with my mother and determined she was depressed and didn't want to be there. My mom was already on an anti-depressant and the one that he prescribed should not have been given in conjunction with the one she was on. In addition, she was having an adverse reaction to the pain medication. She was very sensitive to many pain medications and that is why her primary physician had prescribed the ones that she had. So with these two new medications, my mom was confused, agitated, sleepy and unable to participate in her rehabilitation. I admit that my mother was not happy about being there, but there was no medication that was going to change that. I informed the nurse that I did not want her receiving any more doses of those medications. The nurse informed me that because the doctor had ordered them, they were required to give them. I informed him that my mother had appointed me her Power of Attorney for Heath Care because she felt confident that I could make the appropriate decisions for her, and that designation gave me the right to refuse those medications on her behalf. I eventually went to the manager of the facility explaining not only the chain of command with the Durable Power of Attorney for Health Care, but also my justifications for refusing the medications on my mother's behalf.

Fortunately, in this case I was able to get the facility to honor the designation and follow my wishes. The two things to be gleamed from this story are that you need to be willing to question authority and you need to do your homework in justifying your decisions. Because I was a nurse and possessed the knowledge of my rights afforded by the Durable Power of Attorney for Health Care and knew the pharmacology of the medications involved, I was able to argue my case. This is why it is important to be willing to do your homework and research when acting as someone's Durable Power of Attorney for Health Care. If you do not have the expertise, make sure that you are asking questions, getting second opinions and are willing to follow through to resolution.

Another problem that can crop up occurs when the Durable Power of Attorney for Health Care and the medical providers disagree on the best care options for the patient and things escalate. Health care providers may try to get the designation overturned or ask the courts to get involved to determine whose wishes should be followed. This is why it is important to know your facts, make sure that you are making decisions based on the patient's wishes and not your own personal feelings and try to work cooperatively yet firmly with the patient's health care providers.

Recently, there was a case where the Durable Power of Attorney for Health Care had disagreed with treatment options for a patient she had been working with for months. The health care providers stated that the patient was not incompetent and therefore able to make decisions for herself. The problem was that the patient had just recently suffered a rather significant stroke and was being treated with medications used to slow the progression of dementia. When offered medications by the health care providers, the patient would be agreeable to take the medications, but the Durable Power of Attorney for Health Care, a nurse by profession, felt that the medication was hindering the patient's recovery. The facility threatened to contact the county's family services office. The matter was resolved when the patient was moved to another facility where the health care providers were willing to work with the patient and the Durable Power of Attorney for Health Care.

So the key to the Durable Power of Attorney for Health Care is to pick someone who is familiar with your wishes, willing to go the extra mile in researching the best treatment and willing to stand up for your rights to proper health care treatment. When acting as someone's health care designee, always act in the patient's best interest. If you feel justified in questioning the health care providers involved with the patient's care, then by all means do so respectfully, yet firmly.

DNR

The last medical advance directive that we will look at in this chapter is the DNR order (Do Not Resuscitate). This order by name seems pretty simple, but as with many things in health care, can come packed with many caveats that you need to be aware of before filling out this form for yourself or a person that you have been appointed to make health care decisions for. Once again, this order differs from state to state, so make sure to familiarize yourself with these orders for your state of residence.

Let's look at what the order means. Do Not Resuscitate means that health care providers and/or emergency responders are not to initiate cardiopulmonary resuscitation (CPR) or to insert artificial airways into patients with these designations in writing. If these actions are taken prior to the health care providers being made aware of the designation, they are then to cease any life saving measures that have been initiated once the appropriate documentation has been provided. Do Not Resuscitate does not mean do not treat. There are many treatment options available with this designation.

When would you want to make sure that you have a DNR order signed? Generally, DNR orders are signed toward the end of life because of advanced age, chronic or terminal illness or decreased quality of life.

The order must generally be signed by both the patient or the patient's designated representative and a physician or advanced practice nurse. It is important to make sure that this form is signed by those legally required to sign it in your state. I can't even count how many patients come into the hospital with the order on the chart, but it is not signed by a physician or advanced practice nurse. If the patient intended to be a DNR, those wishes went out the door because no one verified that the appropriate health care provider signed the form.

As stated earlier, in some states these forms are fairly straight forward and state simply that the patient is not to be resuscitated. They may be treated for pain, they may be given oxygen to keep them comfortable and they may be treated for any condition considered to be treatable. They will not have an artificial airway inserted, there will be no CPR and there will be no resuscitative intravenous therapy.

Other states have assigned different levels of treatment options along with the Do Not Resuscitate order. On these forms, the first level that you can check is the line that states that you are a Full Code and desire to have all life saving treatments available. This is sometimes referred to as a Level One Code. The second level can be called a Level Two Code or can also be called a Comfort Care-Arrest. When you select this level, this means that you want to be treated by any means available up until CPR and an artificial airway. This level can cause quite a bit of confusion for not only patients and family members, but also health care providers. The term Comfort Care-Arrest lends to confusion because of the term "Comfort Care". This indicates that the patient only wants comfort care measures taken and no other medical treatment. Many people don't realize that the "Arrest" added on to the end, indicates that treatments up until CPR and artificial airways are allowed. States that have changed this terminology and added it to the Do No Resuscitate forms did so to try to decrease confusion for everyone, but it unfortunately has just created more confusion and debate among health care personnel. The third designation on these forms is the level three code or comfort care. This means that the patient does not want any treatment meant to cure or treat. This designation means that the patient wants comfort care measures only. This can include pain medication, oxygen and in some cases antibiotic therapy, if it is thought that it will increase the patient's comfort.

The important thing to keep in mind when requesting and signing advance directives is to make sure that you understand what the forms are saying and that they are reflective of your desires. If you have questions or trouble understanding the directives, ask several health care providers to explain it to you to make sure that you are getting consistent input and feedback. While advance directives are sometimes confusing, they are vitally important to your health care planning and are documents that all adults should have filled out and available when the occasion arises. If you have residences in more than one state, it is recommended that you have advance directives signed for each state in which you may reside. While most advance directives will cover you during travel, if you spend a significant amount of time in state/states other than your home state, talk to an attorney to see if your advance directives will be honored in all of the states in which you reside.

Legal and Financial Planning

While this book deals mostly in the health care realm, legal and financial planning can often provide for better health care planning, health care resources, and financial health and maintenance. In the next few sections, we will discuss some of the things you should consider and talk to qualified legal and financial professionals about to prevent problems and surprises in the future.

Durable Power of Attorney

This legal document allows you to appoint someone to make financial and legal decisions for you in the event you are unable to make those decisions for yourself. Your legal Durable Power of Attorney and your Durable Power of Attorney for Health Care can be the same person or two different people. For the most appropriate decision in your state of residence, it is best to consult an attorney to see what your best options are. Generally, this is a decision you need to make and a form that you want to have on file before you need it in case of accident, illness or advancing age. The person appointed to this position should be someone whom you trust impeccably as they will, in most states, be able to do everything legally and financially on your behalf.

Guardianships/Conservatorships

In some states these terms are used interchangeably, and in other states there are slight differences between the two. For the purpose of this section, we will use them interchangeably. Guardians are appointed when a person is no longer able to make his own legal, financial and health care decisions. Generally, a guardian is appointed for minors, anyone who is declared mentally incompetent to make their own decisions and often the elderly. Once it is deemed that a person needs a guardian to protect his legal and financial issues, it is generally done through a probate court order. A person can apply to the courts to be named a guardian or, in some cases, the court will appoint a guardian to watch over a person's affairs. A guardian can be a friend, family member or court appointed representative and/ or an attorney. Guardianships can be either permanent or temporary depending on the situation.

While the courts require annual financial reports and review guardianship appointments on an annual basis, there are still abuses that can occur. Many times, it is recommended that you appoint a Durable Power of Attorney to avoid having a guardian appointed for you. If your Durable Power of Attorney takes advantage of the privileges, the court may step in and appoint a guardian to protect your assets.

If you have an elderly loved one and she has appointed you her Durable Power of Attorney, you may at some point need to apply for guardianship. If dementia or Alzheimer's disease comes into play, the person may not be able to make competent decisions and can be easily taken advantage of by others. Unfortunately, we have witnessed many circumstances where a patient has a care giver or someone else that enters her life who does not have her best interest in mind. If the person has not been declared incompetent, they can then sign over their Durable Power of Attorney to another. When someone is able to get a patient to switch appointees, she generally doesn't waste too much time emptying out bank accounts and liquidating assets. To avoid this from happening to the person who has appointed you her Durable Power of Attorney, keep an open line of communication with her health care provider to monitor mental status changes and apply for guardianship before someone else takes advantage of the patient's decreased mental capabilities.

Insurance

Insurance can be a huge part of a well-balanced financial plan. We have talked about how having a health insurance policy can help prevent financial ruin, but there are also many other types of insurance plans on the market that people can purchase to protect themselves and/or their family. When considering purchasing other types of insurance, it is best to talk to a reputable financial planner to see what types of policies will be a benefit for you and your family. Keep in mind, many people in the phone book or found online who advertise themselves as financial planners are selling insurance. It is important to find a financial planner who is not going to benefit financially from selling you a policy.

Life insurance can be an important part of a sound financial plan, especially if you have a spouse/significant other and/or children who depend on your income to make ends meet. If you are single or your children are grown and financially independent, a life insurance policy may not benefit you that much. You may have already purchased a policy that may provide some cash balances that can be used to assist with living or health care costs in the future. A financial planner can help guide you in determining the advantages and disadvantages of the various policies on the market.

The other popular insurance on the market today is Long Term Care insurance. These policies come into play as you age and help cover some of the costs of assisted living and/or skilled nursing care. Where life insurance policies are pretty much a sure bet because eventually we all are going to die, the long term care policies can be a little more of a gamble. Chances are, the majority of us will at some point need some sort of assistance or long term care, but on the other hand, many will never have to use the benefits afforded by these policies. Your decision to buy a policy such as this should, once again, be discussed with a financial planner. These policies can help maintain the value of an estate and can prolong your ability to protect your assets. They can also be quite expensive and, depending on the policy, provide limited coverage. Compare policies and coverages carefully.

There are also disease specific insurance policies on the market. These policies will usually pay out a certain daily amount if you are diagnosed with cancer, heart disease, Alzheimer's, etc. These policies are even more of a gamble. They only pay out if you are diagnosed with the disease named in the policy. Other policies that fall into this category will bill themselves as supplemental policies in case of hospitalization or sickness. Before purchasing these policies, read the small print carefully. Some of these policies will only pay out if you are admitted for a certain number of days and/or in very specific parts of the hospital. Once again, run these policies past a qualified financial planner who is not benefitting from the sales of these policies.

The final types of policies that we will look at are the supplemental health insurance policies that enhance Medicare policies. These policies can help defer some of the medical costs that are not covered by Medicare. They can be offered by employers, the military, hospital systems, retirement organizations and independent health insurance companies. These policies can be helpful, but also require careful reading to see which policy is going to be most beneficial for you.

Wills and Estate Planning

Another part of maintaining your own and your family's financial health is to talk with an estate attorney to see the best way to protect your estate from health care costs and long term care. An attorney can help you plan how to protect your family from financial devastation related to unexpected (or expected) health care costs. We have heard stories of couples who have had to get divorces in order to save a family home or financial assets. To prevent this tragedy, go to an attorney qualified to do estate planning, and just to be sure, get a second opinion as you would with any other major life decision.

Chapter 10

Geriatric Care Management/ Elder Care Planning

Geriatric care management can mean many different things to different people. For some, the term means managing the health, wellness and disease processes of the elderly. To others, it means managing the social, medical, safety and legal concerns of the elderly. For the purpose of this chapter, we will look at many of the above mentioned aspects and how to best navigate the care of the elderly.

Let's first define the term elderly. Many define elderly as 65 years of age and older. Some in the medical profession may define elderly a bit differently, taking into consideration the biological age of a patient versus the chronological age of the patient. So in theory, there may be some patients younger than 65 that may be qualified as elderly based on their biological age and health. On the other hand, you may have someone whose biological age is less than their chronological age and may not be considered part of the elderly category. As we go through this chapter, we will look at the various areas of elder care planning including medical management, living arrangements, social-ization, care concerns and terminology often used in the planning and management of the elderly patient.

Medical Management of the Geriatric Patient

The medical management of the elderly population is often complex and involves many of the body's systems. Many elderly patients are seen by several different specialists, many who don't always communicate with each other. This often leads to what is called polypharmacy.

Polypharmacy is the taking of multiple and many medications. This can involve prescription medications, over-the-counter medications and herbal and dietary supplements. Polypharmacy is not always a bad thing, but can often lead to additional complications in the management of the elderly patient.

Let's first look at some of the advantages of polypharmacy. If an elderly patient has many systems that are diseased or affected by the aging process, medications can control the disease processes and, in some cases, delay progression of disease processes. Medications can lead to improved quality of life and increased longevity. Pharmaceutical management of the aging process can lead to increased independence, pain control and safety.

The disadvantages to polypharmacy can be many and need to be monitored by the patient, medical care providers and family members. As we discussed in earlier chapters, when a patient takes a medication, there may be side effects to that medication that require additional medications. Many patients may experience adverse reactions to the medications that health care providers may interpret as progression of the disease process resulting in additional prescriptions being provided. In addition, the more medications an elderly patient takes, the higher the risk of medication errors such as double dosing or skipped dosing. Of course, cost can be another factor of polypharmacy for the elderly patient. The more medications that the elderly patient is on the greater the financial struggle which often leads to the patient cutting back on his doses and not getting the therapeutic benefits. Many times the patient will be embarrassed to admit that he can't afford his medications and allow his medical care providers to believe that he is taking his medications as prescribed. When the therapeutic benefits are not achieved, the patient's medical provider will often continue to increase the number of medications in an attempt to get control of the disease processes.

People most at risk for the disadvantages of polypharmacy are those patients who are older than 75 years, live alone, have multiple disease processes, decreased mental capacity, decreased vision, decreased dexterity, multiple medical providers and/or take a lot of over-the-counter medications and supplements in addition to their prescription medications without consulting with their health care providers. Many patients often fail to communicate their use of over-the-counter medications and supplements with their health care providers, because they don't think their health care providers will approve or that the over-the-counters don't count.

There are several ways to prevent or at least minimize the negative effects of polypharmacy. First, make sure that there is a primary or family physician involved. Second, make sure that the primary physician is kept informed. The only way to insure that the primary physician is informed is to do it yourself. Specialists, hospitals and extended care facilities do not always update the primary physician, and if they do send something to the primary physician, it is not guaranteed that he will read it. That is why you take your records and updated medication list with you, hand it to your physician personally and discuss it with him in person. Next, make sure that you ask your primary physician to review the medication list and specifically ask if there are any medications that can be eliminated or if there are any medications that may interact with other medications on the list. You can also check with your pharmacist to see if there are medications that may cause problems down the road.

To be even more proactive, you can go to one of the medication interaction web sites and check the interactions yourself. Armed with this information, not only can you ask your health care provider specific questions about the medications you are taking, but also become familiar with side effects, adverse reactions, and drug-to-drug interactions. With this knowledge, you can better ensure the safety of your medications and be familiar with what to expect from the medications. Most of these web sites will have a three tier interaction rating system using a color coding of green, yellow and red. Green means that there are no serious interactions, yellow means there may be some interaction, but the benefits probably outweigh the risks. The red color will represent a warning that a medication may cause a serious interaction with one of your other medications. Yellows and reds are certainly ones that you would want to discuss with your health care provider and pharmacist. Keep in mind, there are times even when a red caution comes up on a medication interaction that the benefits of taking those medications may outweigh the risks, but they still warrant a conversation with your health care provider.

Sensory and memory deficits are other problematic areas in the health maintenance of the geriatric patient. Unfortunately, as we age, our sensory organs start a gradual decline, and in many cases so does our memory capacity. It is difficult for many geriatric patients to hear and totally comprehend what their health care providers are saying to them. It is also difficult for them to read medication labels and educational materials related to their disease management.

To assist the geriatric patient in maintaining safe health care, it is highly recommended that she take someone with her to medical appointments to take notes and be able to repeat important information she may not catch. This is where a health advocate is most important. The person advocating for the patient should have an in-depth knowledge of the patient and her medical history. Optimally, that person should also have at least a basic understanding of medical terminology. Unfortunately, health literacy or lack thereof is something that is often overlooked by health care providers. There are simple tests that the health care provider can perform or that can be found online to guide the health care provider and the advocate in determining a patient's or family member's understanding of health care terminology.

Hearing aids, glasses, large print on prescriptions and educational materials can help insure that the geriatric patient understands and follows medical advice. Unfortunately, many geriatric patients do not like to admit that their sensory organs are failing and will try to cover up these deficits. It is imperative that those involved in the geriatric patient's care, monitor these problems and step up to insure safe medical care. Dealing with memory or comprehension loss can be a little more difficult since there are no mechanical aids that one can purchase to assist with these losses. It is possible to ask the medical provider if they can record the visit to replay later, but some medical providers may object. They shouldn't, but in our litigious society many may balk at the idea. Often if the patient or advocate explains the reasons why, the health care provider may be more sensitive to the recording of the appointment. If as a family member and/or loved one, you sense that the geriatric patient is not able to repeat what happened at her last medical appointment in a manner that makes sense, it may be time to start accompanying her to her appointments or hire someone who understands both the patient and the terminology.

Geriatric Life Management

Managing the life needs of the geriatric patient can be challenging for both the patient and family and friends. In this section, we will discuss some of the lifestyle and life management concerns of the aging patient, provide ideas for implementation of changes that will help to maintain the patient's independence for as long as possible, as well as, provide a greater sense of peace of mind for caregivers and future caregivers.

Driving
Driving is what gives many of us a sense of independence and freedom. The aging patient often finds his driving abilities affected by decreases in sensory abilities such as vision and hearing, decreases in reflexes and reaction times, decreased memory and brain function and increases in chronic health problems. Because driving provides

a strong sense of independence, the older patient may not want to give up the keys. This can create increased stress and worry for those around him, not to mention the other drivers on the road.

When all goes well, the aging patient may realize when her driving abilities are starting to diminish and voluntarily stop driving, but generally there is a lot of discussion and arguing that goes on between the elderly driver and her family before this happens. So when is it time to let someone else do the driving? There is no magic age when everyone should give up driving. There are many people in their nineties who are in very good physical and mental health who are safe drivers, and then there are many people decades younger who are unsafe on the roadways. Below are some suggestions to help in deciding when it is time to let someone else do the driving.

1. Make sure that the older driver has vision, hearing, mental and reflex exams every year.

2. Keep an eye on the condition of the car. Are there a lot of unexplained dents? Are the tires showing signs of wear on the sides indicating a lot of curb riding or misjudging of distances? Is the car being regularly maintained?

3. Monitor the number of accidents and traffic tickets.

4. Does the older driver report having difficulty finding familiar locations?

5. Are neighbors and friends expressing concerns about the patient's driving abilities?

If you have decided that the patient should not be driving, how are you going to convince the patient to hand over the keys and quit driving? Try some of the suggestions below.

1. Start by having a conversation, keeping in mind that you are asking this person to give away a part of his freedom and independence.

Make the conversation as non-threatening as possible and offer alternatives to driving. Alternatives may include a van from the local senior center and/or assistance from friends and family for running errands, doctor appointments and social activities.

2. Sign him up for a senior driving refresher course. This way the department of motor vehicles or agency offering the course can make the appropriate recommendations.

3. Speak with the patient's primary health care provider. Many times, when a doctor speaks to the patient, he tends to listen and follow the advice of the health care provider more so than that of his family and friends. A health care provider can also alert the state's bureau of motor vehicles that the patient is no longer safe to drive and have his driver's license revoked by the state.

4. If you and the patient disagree about the patient's ability to continue driving, make a deal to have the patient go take the driving exam with the results being the deciding factor.

5. When all else fails and there is an imminent danger to the patient driving, you may end up having to take the keys and the car. It is important to remove the temptation. When the car is physically available, I have seen patients call a lock smith or car dealership to get additional keys made and then end up getting lost in other cities or states.

Talking to a loved one about giving up her driving privileges is a stressful event for all involved and needs to be handled delicately. Make sure that you have the facts straight and are doing it for the patient's safety and the safety of others. Offer outings by organizing family and friends to drive the patient where she wants to go. Provide cab or bus passes if the patient is able to safely utilize those modes of transportation. You may also check into various other resources such as church members, social organizations, local hospitals and local social services agencies. Be delicate, but remain firm.

Living Arrangements
Once an aging patient loses his ability to safely drive, his independence is greatly diminished. Deciding when to give up the family home, condo or apartment is a very individual process. There are many alternatives to consider depending on the person, health status, financial health and support network. In this section we will look at the various options available to the aging patient, methods to prolong independence and the steps involved in making the right decisions for optimal outcomes.

Staying in the Home

Staying in the home is the preferred choice of most people as they age. The home is a place where people feel secure, they have their possessions around them that can provide comfort and it is an environment that they have tailored to their wants and needs. The goal of most elders and their children is to keep the elder in that home for as long as possible. Let's look at several key factors when deciding how long to stay in the home.

1. The home should be safe for the occupants. Safety includes making sure that the home is well maintained, the mechanicals are in good working order and the surrounding neighborhood should have a relatively good safety record. In addition, the home should be elder-proofed. Elder-proofing a home should include making sure that all hand rails and grab bars are secure. The home should be free from clutter and provide roomy walkways. Items that are used on a regular basis should be within reach so that the resident doesn't have to use ladders or step stools to reach things that he uses frequently. Laundry areas should be on the main level to avoid increased risks of falling down steps. Lighting inside and out should be adequate for good visualization and safety. In colder climates, the outside areas should be free of ice and snow. Bathrooms should be equipped with grab bars and skid free surfaces. Rugs and floorings

should be secure to prevent tripping and falls. The home should also be equipped with a security system with a medical alert service in case of falls or an inability to get to the phone.

2. The resident should have access to transportation. If she is no longer able to drive, make sure that there is a good supply of family and friends to meet the resident's transportation needs. Look into community services that may provide safe and affordable transportation. If the elder is no longer able to drive, make sure that the car is removed from the property. Sometimes the temptation for independence is too great. Remember removing keys is not much of a deterrent to someone determined to drive.

3. The elder resident should have access to socialization. Many elders start to suffer increased depression, withdrawal and decreased health maintenance when they do not get enough socialization. Try to find activities that they are interested in and then make sure that they have access and transportation to those activities. Encourage other family members and friends to call and drop in for visits. The more stimulation the mind gets, the sharper it will stay, the risk of depression will be lessened and the more their health will be maintained.

4. Make sure that there is an ability to obtain adequate nutrition. Many times, the elderly lose interest in making meals or are physically unable. Vision problems make reading recipes difficult. Joint pain can make standing in the kitchen a painful experience. Taste buds are not as sharp as they once were and appetite is negatively impacted. Sometimes cost is a factor in obtaining nutritious foods. Once again, have family and friends take turns making meals or taking them out to eat.

5. Keep an eye on their health maintenance and ability to take their medications as prescribed. Keep track of doctor's appointments and make sure that transportation is available. Are they suffering symptoms that are related to taking too much or too little of their prescribed medication? Ask about the use of over-the-counter

medications to make sure that they are taking them as intended.

6. Look for any signs of financial struggles. Unopened or unpaid bills lying around the house are a sign that the elder is having financial troubles or problems keeping up with the process. Look for large bank withdrawals. Many times the elderly population is targeted by a variety of scam artists. Be leery of new friendships accompanied by a decrease in the bank account. Listen closely if the aging person starts to complain about the bank making mistakes and her accounts being out of balance. Once you identify that there is a problem, it may be time to have a discussion about a trusted family member or friend helping with the accounts. If the problem is getting really severe, then it is time to talk to an attorney about the best options for the individual situation.

What Happens Next?

There often comes a time when you have done everything possible to keep the elder in her own home and independent, and the problems keep mounting. How do you know when it is time to take the next step?

Answering the following questions and heeding the following warnings may help in taking that next step.

1. Are there frequent falls, unexplained bruises, cuts or burns? This may indicate that the patient is having difficulty navigating the home environment. The solution is to elder proof the home by modifying bathrooms, kitchens, floor coverings, steps and hand railings. Have the patient assessed for ambulatory aids such as canes, walkers and/or scooter chairs.

2. Is the patient losing weight and experiencing a lot of food spoilage? The solution is to see if the patient qualifies for community services

that deliver meals to the home or takes the patient out for meals on a daily basis. Many of these programs are low cost or free depending on the community service and the financial status of the patient.

3. Are health problems and disease management being impacted by inconsistent medication management? The solution is to set up a weekly medication box and check it frequently. If the patient is demonstrating a decrease in mental capacity, it may be more beneficial to only fill up one day at a time. There have been stories where caregivers have set up a med box for a week and instructed the patient to make sure he takes all of his medications, just to find that he took all seven days in one day. It also helps to obtain a medication watch to remind him of the times of day that he should be taking his medications. If all else fails, it may become necessary to have a family member or paid caregiver stop in several times a day to insure adherence to the medication schedule.

4. Are there signs of decreased hygiene? The solution is to have someone come in and offer assistance for bathing and laundry. Once again, it may be possible to tap into community care giving services or hire a home health aide service.

5. Are there noticeable changes in the patient's finances? Often the elderly patient falls victim to home repair scams, mail order offers, telephone scams and internet scams. The solution to this problem is to talk with the patient about appointing a Power of Attorney or guardian to oversee the patient's finances. This often involves removing credit cards and checkbooks from the premises so that the temptation is removed.

6. Are things just totally getting out of hand and you feel the patient's health and safety is at risk? If the goal at this point is to still allow the patient to remain in her own home, then you may have to look at moving someone in to provide around the clock supervision of the patient. If this should be the case, it can be a family member, friend or professional caregiver. It is important to keep in mind

that vigilance is still required to prevent the live-in care giver from taking advantage and unduly influencing the patient into harmful financial and legal moves.

There are times when it becomes increasingly difficult to accommodate keeping the patient in his own home. Sometimes the burden on the family becomes too much, and the health and welfare of both the family caregiver and the patient are put in jeopardy despite the best of intentions. Before this happens, it may be worthwhile to look at some of the other alternatives. Some of the alternatives mentioned below may be considered very early in the process. We will discuss the alternatives and some of their advantages and disadvantages as we go.

1. Downsizing – Downsizing is one of the first moves we make as we age. The living space gets smaller and is generally a one level floor plan. This can accommodate a change in lifestyle as people try to cut costs into retirement, decrease their level of work around the house and simplify their life on all levels. The advantage to downsizing is that it can often increase the longevity of independence. The simpler the surroundings, the longer you are able to maintain your environment. There are very few disadvantages to downsizing. There are some people who suffer separation anxiety from parting with some of their belongings. There are new companies sprouting up around the country to help people deal with these anxieties. These companies will come in and delicately help to decide what to keep, what to donate, what to trash and what to sell. The other disadvantage for some is that they lose some of their sense of purpose and are not quite sure what to do without a house and yard to maintain.

2. Retirement Communities – Retirement communities often offer an opportunity to downsize around people of similar age and similar interests. Some retirement communities also offer other facilities to accommodate further downsizing or increased health care needs. This allows the person to stay in a community where she is comfortable and where her friends are close by. The advantage of the retirement community is that you can

still maintain a high degree of independence, because many of these communities provide services such as shuttles, communal meals, and scheduled activities. When picking a community, it is important to select one that has people of similar ages, interests and comparable levels of health. A disadvantage to these communities is they can be more expensive. There are some retirement communities that provide income based pricing that are less expensive. The other disadvantage is that if you pick a community that consists of people who are substantially older, younger or in better or worse health than you, you run the risk of greater isolation and depression.

3. Assisted Living Facilities – Assisted living facilities are another option when a patient's care needs increase. Many assisted living facilities offer private rooms and apartments along with assistance with daily activities, meals and medical care. Most assisted living facilities offer different levels of assistance based on the individual's needs. The cost, of course, goes up as additional assistance is needed. The advantages of these facilities are that they provide a sense of independence while helping manage disease processes and medication regimes. These facilities can be rather costly, but some of the costs can be covered by long term care insurance. In some cases, there are also veteran's benefits available to assist with the cost. The requirement to qualify for these benefits is based on income and having served in the military during wartime. The main disadvantage to assisted living facilities is generally the cost. They can range in cost from 2,000 dollars a month and up.

4. Nursing Homes – Nursing homes are often the places that most people want to avoid, but they can be a life saver to both patient and family members. These facilities generally provide a home for those who have chronic health problems, are unable to live independently and can't afford the assisted living route, as well as people who have advanced in their level of care to the extent that their family and friends can longer provide for their care. The advantages to nursing homes are that they specialize

in total nursing care and generally have a full medical staff available 24 hours a day. The disadvantages are that they can be very expensive, and it is sometimes difficult to find one that provides the level of care that you wish for your loved one.

5. Specialized Care Facilities – There are facilities that specialize in certain diseases such as Alzheimer's disease, stroke rehabilitation, hospice, etc. These facilities are very good for patients with specific diagnoses. The advantage of these types of facilities is the staff is generally highly trained in dealing with the specified disease and can increase and extend the patient's quality of life. The disadvantage once again can, in most cases, be cost.

Deciding what type of living arrangement is going to be best can be a complex process. The patient's wishes should be the first consideration. Many times family members will want to keep the patient at home at all costs. While this may work in some circumstances where there is a large support network in place, other times it leads to the patient becoming isolated. The other problem is care giver burnout. Caring fulltime for a family member or loved one is an all consuming activity and comes with a great deal of stress. Even when family care givers have medical training, it can be difficult at best. When care giver stress increases, so does the risk of abuse and neglect.

Overall, the management of the geriatric patient can be stressful for both the patient and the care giver. The goal is to manage things in such a way as to maintain the highest quality of life for all involved. Because geriatric care management of a loved one can be an emotional issue for all involved, it is important to tap into as many resources as possible. These resources can be found in many places including health care facilities, governmental agencies, non-profit agencies, libraries, senior centers, churches, neighborhood organizations, counseling centers, as well as with friends and families. At some point, it may be worth consulting with an independent geriatric care manager or health advocate to do the research for you to make sure that you and your loved are getting the help and services available to help maintain quality of life throughout the geriatric life span.

Chapter 11

Advocating to the End

Advocating for a loved one is a job that lasts to the end. The end of life is fraught with many emotions and challenges and, as stated in earlier chapters, having discussions with loved ones about end of life issues paves the way for an easier transition for all involved. When you have had these important discussions with your loved ones, it makes the decision making process easier, it eases guilt and it gives you a sense of control and strength to help each other through life's final transition.

Watching a loved one's health decline is perhaps one of the hardest things to witness. When that loved one is no longer able to make decisions regarding his own health care, the decisions are going to be up to you or perhaps another family member. Many times these decisions will be intertwined with family history, religious/spiritual beliefs and medical terminology. As we go through this chapter, we will focus the discussion on how to make the most appropriate medical decisions through the end stages of life.

It is said that the majority of a patient's lifetime medical costs occurs within the last two weeks of her life. So what that means is that we are spending a lot of money to prolong life for two weeks. Of course, when we are talking about our loved ones, we don't like to think about putting a price tag on that life. It is unfortunate, but at some point all of us, as health care consumers, need to start thinking about this to a certain extent and act responsibly. Not only do we need to think about our social responsibility, but we must also think about what processes we are often putting our loved ones through during their last days of life.

Making the right decisions for a loved one at the end of life is a huge responsibility, and there is no single right answer for every situation. Each individual's life will end in a very unique and personal way. As an advocate for a loved one, it will be up to you call the shots. To do this will require information regarding health status, prognosis, quality of life, personal wishes, family dynamics and religious and spiritual beliefs. As we go through this chapter, we will look at all of the issues that get factored in to end of life decisions as well as look at some stories that may help illustrate how to work through the decision making process.

Health Status and Prognosis

The health status of the patient is, of course, a major factor in determining when to end medical treatment. The younger the patient, the harder it is to make the decision to stop aggressive medical care. The overall health status of the patient is one guide in making the determination. Asking yourself several questions will help you make it through the decision making process.

1. Has the patient battled a chronic illness for a long period of time? The longer the patient has fought an illness, the fewer reserves he has to keep fighting. If he has been fighting for a long period of time and has a poor prognosis and a poor quality of life, then it may be time to consider ending aggressive treatment.

2. Has the patient suffered a severe traumatic injury? There have been great advances in the treatment of traumatic injuries and people are not only surviving, but returning to a fairly high quality of life. However, there are many times when the injuries are just too severe. At this point, it is important to have a serious conversation with the patient's health care providers to determine long term prognosis and quality of life. It is important that you initiate

these discussions, because many times health care providers will not address them and continue to provide aggressive treatment knowing that the treatment in the end will most likely be futile. Remember, these are very difficult discussions for all involved, and many health care providers will be hesitant to approach you with end of life decisions.

As stated earlier, the age of the patient also plays into the decision. The younger the age, the more a prolonged and aggressive treatment regime might be justified. The older we get, the chances of surviving a major health crisis decreases proportionately. The ability of the elderly patient to recover is decreased due to the toll of chronic illnesses, decreased nutrition and degeneration of the major organ systems. While it is possible to extend life in even the oldest patients, it is often painful and traumatic to the patient. Once again, have a discussion with the health care providers. Ask as many questions as you need to in order to make an informed decision and be prepared to hear what the health care provider is saying.

Let's look at a couple of different scenarios and how the decisions were made in regard to treatment options and end of life decisions. The first scenario I will use happened to involve my own mother. She was 91 years old and in relatively good health, both mentally and physically. Her main problem was she suffered from rather significant arthritis and degenerative joint disease. These afflictions caused her a great deal of daily pain. The pain was kept mostly in check with prescription anti-inflammatory medications. She had started to verbalize things such as, "Why do you have to live so long and be so miserable." Eventually, the pain got so bad she could not get out of bed. We took her to the hospital for pain control. The x-rays that were done showed she was bone on bone in both her knee and hip.

My mother had gotten to the point where she could no longer stand up on her own, and just lying in bed was causing excruciating pain and muscle spasms. I had a long conversation with the orthopedic surgeon who initially stated that doing a double joint replacement on a 91-year- old was probably not the greatest of ideas. On a medical level, I agreed with him knowing that a surgery of that magnitude came with many potential complications. The other option was to keep her heavily medicated with narcotic pain medications which rendered her basically unresponsive and would result in moving her into a nursing home. Considering that she was still very mentally aware and in relatively good physical health, I could not think of her being either in unbearable pain or unresponsive. Consequently, I had a discussion with my mom about the options, and she opted for the surgery. I went back to the surgeon and discussed the surgery with him. At this point, he stated that if her bones were broken we would not think twice about fixing them, so we might as well proceed with the surgery.

After the decision was made, my mother started running a high fever and subsequent blood tests showed a massive infection in her bloodstream that was caused by her IV site. While we waited for the results of the blood tests, my mother had started going into multiple organ failure. Her family physician stated that they could try a very high powered antibiotic to fight the infection, but the antibiotic itself would put additional stress on her vital organs. Without antibiotic therapy, she would pass away in two days. After a discussion with her family physician, it was decided that we would medicate her for comfort and let the infection run its course. This was a very difficult decision for me to make, as a daughter, regarding my mother and last living family member. As a nurse and a daughter, I realized that her chances for a complete recovery were very minimal. We still had the problem of the hip and knee pain and with the infection surgery was no longer an option, at least not for quite some time. While waiting for the infection to clear, she would have received high doses of pain medications which would bring a higher risk of pneumonia, skin breakdown and continued suffering. At this point, I felt comfortable that I had made the right decision, and her physician agreed.

Having made the decision not to treat the infection, her physician turned her care over to a palliative physician for comfort care measures and pain management. This is where the story takes a turn that trips many family members up when making medical decisions for loved ones. The palliative physician called me to tell me that he

was going to order a CT scan of my mother's abdomen. Now having
made the decision to procede with comfort care measures, I was
puzzled as to why he would want to do a scan. First, there had been
absolutely no indication that she was having any abdominal issues.
Second, we had determined that the source of infection was from the
IV site. He then told me that when he felt her belly during his assessment, my mother winced in pain. I asked him if the pain was on the
right side of her abdomen when she winced. He stated that indeed
it was. I informed him that I felt her wincing was from her right hip
pain which would have been affected by pressing on the right side of
her abdomen. I knew that even when I accidentally bumped the bed
when visiting her, she winced in pain from the slightest movement of
the bed. I then asked this physician why he would even propose such
a thing. Had he not read her family physician's notes stating that we
had decided to provide comfort care only?

I found this action on his part extremely insensitive and bordering on
unethical. After all, I had spent a great deal of time making this decision and felt that now he was questioning that decision. I remember
asking him if he was the palliative physician and was it not his job to
support my decision and direct the comfort care measures. In addition, he had changed her medications against my wishes resulting
in increased pain and discomfort for my mother. Needless to say, I
fired him within six hours of being on the case and requested that her
family physician manage her care to the end.

Unfortunately, many families are faced with these kinds of decisions and if there are multiple family members involved in the decision making process, actions such as the ones taken by the palliative
physician can cause great disconcert among the family and prolonged
suffering for the patient. In this case, was the palliative physician's
desire to do a CT scan an attempt to truly help my mother, poor
assessment skills, an attempt to protect himself from a lawsuit, or
an opportunity to rack up more bills? Frankly, I am not sure what
his motivation was, but it, at least momentarily, made me doubt my
decision.

Let's look at another scenario our company handled. The patient was a gentleman in his early 80's who lived with his wife in their own home. He had a medical history of cardiac disease with bypass surgery and stroke. He suddenly came down with what everyone thought was a bad cold. After his symptoms progressed, he went to the emergency room and was diagnosed with pneumonia. It was decided that he could be discharged home and treated with oral antibiotics. This was the first error in judgment by his health care providers. A patient with his history and diagnosis should have been admitted for IV antibiotic therapy. His condition worsened at home and he was taken back to the hospital and admitted with pneumonia and had subsequently developed blood clots in the lungs. After several days of treatment, his health care providers made the second bad decision. The patient was discharged to an assisted living facility for rehabilitation. This discharge came despite his wife protesting and requesting additional time in the hospital for continued medical care. The patient arrived at the assisted living facility and quickly developed increased difficulty breathing. His wife had repeatedly brought his increased difficulty breathing to the attention of the nursing and medical staff. They told her that the patient's symptoms should be expected and to not worry. At this point, the wife called our company for help and guidance. The presentation that the wife described was one of congestive heart failure. This was not surprising considering that the patient had a rather considerable cardiac history, and his body and cardiac system were being stressed by the pneumonia and blood clots in his lungs.

After the call from the wife, I placed a call to the assisted living facility and asked to talk to the nurse taking care of the patient. I explained who I was and what my concerns were. The nurse was not familiar with the patient's medical history and stated that the doctor had been in just two hours earlier and said everything was fine. I explained to her that the wife was quite concerned and it would be greatly appreciated if she would go and reassess the patient and call me back. When the nurse called back, she stated that the patient was being transported to the hospital.

Prior to the start of this illness, the patient had stated to his wife that he did not desire to be resuscitated as his quality of life had declined over the last several years. While the patient had verbalized these wishes, there had never been a Do Not Resuscitate order written. I advised the wife that she had to initiate this at the hospital because based on his reported presentation it was quite possible that the physicians in the emergency department may put him on a ventilator. When she arrived at the emergency department, she instructed the ER physician to write the DNR order. The patient's heart was quite stressed and his prognosis was not good. In the following days, the wife rallied the family to the hospital and there were many discussions on how to proceed with treatment. It was at this point that I provided the patient and the family with extensive education about the disease processes that were taking their toll on the patient. The patient and the family were able to express their wishes to the medical care providers with a lot more confidence and comfort. The patient did pass away about three days after returning to the hospital, but he was kept comfortable, his family members were all able to make it to the hospital while he was still coherent, and the end came peacefully for all. There were no heroic attempts at prolonging the life beyond what this patient and his body decided was the right time.

The last example we will look at, was a case that happened in the hospital setting. An advocate would have been very useful to the family in this case. An elderly man who had several chronic health problems was brought to the emergency room by ambulance. The patient had a long history of diabetes with complications. He had suffered a stroke that had left him unresponsive. He had both legs amputated above the knee from complications from the diabetes. He had a breathing tube and feeding tube as a result of the stroke. He also was in the late stages of dementia, deaf and blind. Shortly after arriving in the emergency room, the patient went into cardiac arrest. His paper work stated that he was to have full resuscitative measures activated in the event of a cardiac arrest. The medical providers talked with the family members to insure that this was what they truly wanted, considering the patient's condition. The family stated that yes they did indeed want all life saving measures taken. The staff in the room all felt that this was a huge disservice to the patient whose quality of life was so poor. The staff also wanted to respect the family's wishes. In the end, the staff ran a very non-aggressive code. The family was outside the room and felt that all measures had been taken, and the staff made sure that the patient was treated with respect and kept comfortable throughout the process. There were no deep compressions, no unnecessary needle sticks and no additional breathing tubes put down his throat.

Was what the staff did in this situation ethical? Well, that could be debated endlessly by medical ethicists and spiritual leaders. The fact was this patient had an immensely poor quality of life. The family perhaps was hanging on to memories of what the patient used to be or perhaps had unrealistic hopes of what the patient could be. In this case, the staff felt that they allowed the patient to die with dignity while allowing the family to believe that all had been done.

There are many beliefs and arguments regarding end of life issues. There are those who believe absolutely everything should be done to preserve life regardless of age and prognosis, and others who believe in letting nature take its course. When you are faced with making these decisions for a loved one, your religious/spiritual beliefs will come into play. There may also be other family members whose beliefs differ from yours and/or the patient's, and they will want their wishes heard. Knowing and following the patient's wishes should always be the first priority and concern. If you were not able to have those discussions with the patient, then you have to follow the path you believe that the patient would want. Hopefully, you will have some idea as to the patient's wishes, his quality of life and his spiritual beliefs.

Problems usually crop up when too many family members get involved in the decision making process. Each family member may have very different opinions on how to proceed. When this happens, it is sometimes helpful to bring in a neutral party to aid in bringing things to a peaceful resolution. The neutral party may be a hospital chaplain, the patient's primary care giver, a family spiritual adviser, a Hospice program representative, a health advocate or a person knowledgeable of the patient's life and desires. The best results are more frequently achieved when all family members are in agreement. It is important when coming to terms with end of life decisions that family members set aside, as much as possible, any pre-existing family disagreements and jealousies.

As mentioned above, one source that can help patients and families deal with end of life issues is a Hospice organization. Hospice employees are specially trained to deal with end of life issues. A good Hospice service will help the patient with pain control, accepting terms of her life and death and will help the family through the transition. There are both for profit and non-profit Hospice organizations that can provide help to everyone. It is important to remember that Hospice does not promote death nor do they do anything to hasten death, but rather provide support and guidance through the end of life process. There are times when Hospice is called into to help a patient and the patient and/or her body decide that it is not time. If the patient's health rebounds, Hospice will halt their services until the patient and family decide that those services are needed again.

At the end, it can be difficult to watch your loved one pass. Once again, each patient and family member will have different ways of dealing with the actual death. I have seen patients in the hospital setting wait for a family member to arrive from another state before passing. I have also seen family members waiting and wanting to be with a patient when he took his last breath, and the patient passes shortly after the family members have left to get something to eat. It seems that the patient in these cases will be the one calling the shots, and as a family member, you should not feel excessive guilt for not being there at the end. Chances are that was the patient's plan.

Quality of Life and personal Choice

Quality of life is a very subjective topic. One person may look at a situation and say that the quality of life is poor and another may see it as tolerable and make the best of the situation. As an advocate for a loved one, it is important to respect the patient's definition of quality of life. It is natural to want to prolong the life of someone who is important in your life, but once again, try to put your personal feelings aside and make your decision based on the patient's expression of quality of life.

So what determines quality of life? Can the patient still participate in the activities that he has enjoyed throughout his life? Is the patient able to enjoy the company of others? Is the patient experiencing significant and chronic pain? Does the patient spend most of his day sleeping? Has the patient started to show signs of nutritional decline? Is the patient mentally alert and oriented? Does the patient appear to be afraid or paranoid of family, friends and caregivers?

Answering these questions will help to decide a patient's quality of life and help to guide medical care. Let's look at an example. The patient suffers from Alzheimer's disease which has progressed significantly. The patient no longer recognizes loved ones, can no longer participate in familiar activities, and shows little interest in eating. It may be determined that this patient's quality of life is minimal. So what does this mean for the patient's medical management? Certainly as an advocate for this patient, you would want to make sure that she is kept comfortable and that pain is kept to a minimum. Now let's say that it is discovered during a routine medical appointment that the patient has a lump in her breast. As an advocate, what would be your next move?

Undoubtedly, the medical care provider may recommend further diagnostic testing. As an advocate, you may want to ask yourself and the medical provider why. The patient has already been diagnosed with a progressive disease process that is not going to get any better. Treating the cancer aggressively can cause the patient additional pain and suffering. Allowing the cancer to progress may or may not cause additional pain or suffering. Many breast cancers diagnosed late in life tend to be very slow growing and may never bother the patient in her natural lifetime. If allowed to go untreated, any symptoms that may be experienced by the patient can be managed to insure comfort. Based on this line of thinking, why would you consider additional diagnostic testing? Perhaps the medical care provider wants to see how aggressive the cancer is. Your decision should be based on your knowledge of the patient and honest information obtained from extensive questioning of the medical care provider.

Family Dynamics

Family dynamics can be as individual as patients themselves and can be a huge factor when advocating for a loved one. It behooves the patient if all family members work together and are on the same page, but this unfortunately is not always the case. In many situations, the family member who is the primary care giver is not the same person who is designated legally responsible for the patient. In these situations, we will often see disagreements and opposition between the care giver and the power of attorney. In these circumstances, the care giver either lives with or near the patient, and the power of attorney in a different location. The care giver, who has the most knowledge and time invested in the patient's care, has to follow the directives of the legal representative. Issues arise when the legal representative does not have an understanding of the patient's medical and physical needs and may deny employing additional help, make medical decisions that are not in the best interest of the patient or put the care giver through numerous hoops in providing and guiding the care of the patient.

These situations develop for a number of reasons. In some families, the oldest child is often made the legal representative regardless of the physical proximity to the patient. In other cases, some family members may be determined to be more trustworthy in regards to legal and financial matters, but once again do not live close enough to provide regular supervision of care. When this is the case, it is important to put hurt feelings aside, keep an open line of communication and work toward reaching the decisions that are most appropriate for the patient.

In some instances, it may be appropriate to appoint the care giver as the health care power of attorney and another family member the legal power of attorney.

The other way that family dynamics can interfere with the proper advocating of a patient's health care, involves unresolved personal issues. In these situations, family members often try to prolong the life of the patient due to the unresolved issues, wanting just a little bit longer to make up for the lost time or to try to have more time for resolution. The best advice to avoid this issue is to work on these resolutions before it's too late. Sometimes seeking counsel from another family member, friend or adviser can help the family member work through the issue in order to act in the patient's best interest.

Watching a loved one go through the end of life process can be an emotionally draining experience for all involved. To avoid these situations and lessen the stress, try to resolve as many issues as possible as they arise and before it is too late. If issues do come up, and they probably will, try to seek feedback from a neutral party and remember to act in the best interest of the patient and according to the patient's wishes.

Spiritual and Religious Considerations

This is another area that can cause turmoil during the end of life process. Even in families that practice the same religion, there may be different interpretations on what constitutes the will of the source of worship. In Christianity for example, one family member may think that it is God's will to prolong life by all means available, thinking that God provided for creation of the many life saving measures. Another member of the family may think that many of the modern medical interventions are taking God's place and are against God's will. These are very difficult issues to resolve because a person's spiritual beliefs are deeply rooted, and each person is going to insist that his belief is most correct. To resolve these issues, it is sometimes helpful to seek the counsel of a trusted religious leader that can perhaps find common ground and compromises for the family members.

The other area where spiritual and religious beliefs can come into play during end of life process is when the medical interventions are in direct conflict with the edicts of the religion. Most hospitals and care facilities try to work with patients and families within the patient and family's belief system. If you find that the facility is not respecting your religious and or spiritual beliefs, you may request to speak with the facility's ethics board or ask a leader from your place of worship to speak with the facility's management. In the worst case scenario, some facilities will take the issue to court, but this is rare and generally surrounds medical decisions involving children.

After the End
When the patient has passed on and you were the one advocating for the patient, you will no doubt have a period of second guessing yourself. You will go over the decisions that you made for the patient and ask yourself if you made the right decisions. This is a typical care giver response. At this point, you have to trust that you did everything you could with the information that you had available. As long as your decisions were made according to the patient's wishes and in the patient's best interest, then you did all that you could have done. In the end, there is only so much you can do and you must give yourself credit for being there when the patient needed you. When a loved one dies you will enter into a very normal pattern of grief. This grief can last up to two years. Grief is normal and tough to navigate, but remember not to add to the grief with second guessing and post decisional regrets.

Speaking of the grief process, it is important to realize that each person will express grief in his own way. Some people are very comfortable expressing their grief publicly, while others may find visible displays of grief difficult, if not impossible. How someone shows his grief is not necessarily a reflection of the depth of his sadness. A person who is uncomfortable expressing his emotions, may never be seen showing an outward sign of grief such as crying. It is advisable not to judge the depth of someone's sadness by outward expressions.

People will also go through the long term grief process in different ways. Some family members may want to quickly wrap up the details following a loved one's death. They will want to clean out closets, close out financial matters, and sell property as if erasing any visible memory of the deceased. Other family members may not be able to undertake these tasks for a longer period of time. There is no right or wrong way, but compromises may have to be struck in order to keep all family members happy and involved. When conflict arises, it is again advisable to turn to neutral parties, religious or spiritual advisers and/or counselors to make sure the needs of those left behind are addressed.

While advocating for a patient at the end of life can be stressful, thankless and tiring, it can also be rewarding and soothing to know you were there for the patient when she most needed someone to speak on her behalf. Allow yourself time to review the many positive things that you did on the patient's behalf and make sure that you appoint someone that can advocate for you until the end.

Chapter 12

What to Expect in the Future

The future of health care is going to be ever changing. Some of those changes will be beneficial and others may leave us wondering what happened. Health care reform will be debated, changed, debated and changed again and again. Eventually, everyone will have to make tough decisions including individuals, governments and the medical profession. Everyone will have to accept increased responsibility and integrity if health care accessibility is to become favorable for all.

When looking at the various aspects of some of the newest reform possibilities, the changes will impact everyone. As politicians and advocacy groups work toward health coverage and access for everyone, the health care field will continue to become more overwhelmed. There will continue to be debate over whether health care is a basic right for all human beings. It would no doubt take another book to deal with and discuss the complexities of these issues. No matter what your beliefs or opinions on this topic are, there will be a future influx of people needing an increasing amount of health care services. This, of course, is due to a large number of factors we have touched on, such as people living longer, the economy and population growth.

It will take time to prepare the doctors, advanced practice professionals and nurses to handle the increased influx of patients. If more people have insurance and access to health care, there will be longer wait times to see a medical care provider, longer wait times for procedures and changes to the type of care offered. On the plus side, more people will be better able to seek preventive care and screenings thereby catching disease processes in their earlier stages when they are easier and cheaper to treat.

There are already changes that are taking place that you will, no doubt, see more of in the future. Let's take a look at just a few of them:

1. Increased use of advanced practice personnel. – Advanced practice personnel include nurse practitioners and physician assistants. These professions will start seeing more of the patients while physicians will be managers of mass numbers of patients and will only see the sickest of the sick. The advantage of using advanced practice personnel, is they can be trained in less time and placed into the marketplace much sooner than physicians. That can also be the disadvantage. Professionals with less training, will be managing a population that is older and sicker than we have ever seen in the past.

Right now, the numbers of advanced practice personnel is increasing and, for the most part, have received good reviews from patients. The comment heard from many patients is that the advanced practice personnel generally spend more time with them, are better at and have more time to provide patients with education on disease and health management. As long as the supply keeps up with the demand, this can be another positive for the use of advanced practice personnel. If supply does not keep up, then the advanced practice personnel will have less time and will be moving patients in and out at the same rate many doctors do now. The downside is that many of these professionals do not receive the amount of diagnostic training that physicians do and may not be as capable of catching some disease processes.

As a patient, it will be up to you to decide whether or not you feel comfortable seeing an advanced practice professional, but keep in mind that you will have an increasingly difficult time getting into see a physician. Give these professionals a chance, and then if you

do not feel comfortable, have a discussion with the supervising
physician or find another practice where physician services are
more readily available. My personal experience related to advanced
practice personnel has been positive, especially in the emergency
room setting. These professionals can handle many types of health
care concerns, allowing more patients to be seen and allowing the
physicians more time to focus on proper care management of the
patient population.

2. Increased use of less trained ancillary staff. – The ancillary staff
   in the health care setting includes positions such as technicians,
   nurses' aides and medication aides. These positions often employ
   people with minimal to no training in health care. This group
   of personnel is generally less expensive to train and to employ.
   The increased use of ancillary personnel can be related to the
   nationwide nursing shortage and the increased cost of health care
   delivery. In order to lessen the workload on the number of practicing nurses, health care facilities have started to rely on the
   ancillary staff to pick up the slack. Once again, the advantage here
   is that there are more people helping to take care of patients. The
   disadvantage is that these personnel are being given more and
   more responsibility with very little additional training. While in
   some areas the use of these personnel is a necessity to meet the
   patient demands, in other areas it is a cost saving for the facility's
   bottom line. The one area that concerns me is the use of medication aides. This is an area where a few hours of training are just
   not enough. We are seeing an increased number of patients in
   long-term care facilities, facilities that employ the majority of
   these aides, coming into the hospital system with problems directly
   related to improper medication practices. As a patient or an advocate for a patient, it is going to be up to you to make sure the medications are being administered properly. Do not be afraid to ask
   questions, and expect the person administering the medications to
   have the appropriate knowledge of the medications that they are
   administering.

The use of ancillary personnel has been vexing to the general public. Many patients and family members assume that everyone who walks into their room is a nurse. This is often not the case, especially in doctors' offices. Many physicians no longer employ registered nurses unless it is the position of an office manager. If you have a question about the skills and qualifications of anyone taking care of you, by all means, ask. If the answer you get is not the one you want, make your feelings known. Many health care facilities are now making it easier to identify nurses by putting the letters RN in bigger letters on identification badges. If you do not see this indication, it will probably behoove you to ask the person about their training and qualifications.

3. Concierge Medicine – Concierge medicine is a new trend that doctors are discovering. It is a method of insuring a consistent income and giving patients who can afford it, a dedicated doctor. The principle behind concierge medicine is that a doctor agrees to limit the number of patients that she accepts into her practice. Those patients pay fees, which range generally in the thousands of dollars per year, to insure that they will be able to get an appointment within a reasonable amount of time and be able to spend a longer amount of time with the physician. These fees only cover the privilege of being a patient of that physician. All tests, labs, medications and consultations are either covered by the patient or the patient's insurance. These physicians, for the most part, do not do any billing to the insurance companies. They will send any associated bills to the patient, and the patient is responsible for getting any compensation that may be available through their insurance coverage.

Patients who have participated in concierge medicine express satisfaction with the arrangement. Many doctors will include home visits as part of their concierge services, so who wouldn't be happy? The advantages to concierge medicine, of course, are that physicians have the ability to spend more time with patients, provide quicker service, have more time for education, health and disease management and probably provide better service than most of us are accustomed to receiving.

There are disadvantages to concierge medicine. If we look at this service from a more global perspective, we can see that the one major disadvantage is the more doctors who take this direction, the more doctors who are being taken out of the mainstream of availability to the general patient population. It is going to become an even bigger pay to play arena than we currently have. This is a win-win situation for doctors and for patients who can afford these services. The doctors have a guaranteed income, they usually experience a decrease in workload and hours worked, and they no longer have to worry about dealing with the insurance companies. Patients who can't afford these services will have fewer doctors to choose from, longer wait times and spend less time with the doctor. The other disadvantage that may surface is if patients are paying for the privilege of their own personal doctor, will doctors feel additional pressure to give the patient what they want versus what they need? Because this practice is still relatively new, there is not a lot of research or information on how these pay to play relationships will affect medical care and what influence they will have on doctors' practices.

My medical crystal ball tells me the more popular this practice becomes, the more the government will see a need to start regulating this option. With an increased emphasis on health care reform, affordable health care and a deficit of health care providers, the practice of concierge medicine is going to throw a wrench in the plan to provide care for the masses at a reasonable cost. On the other side of my medical crystal ball, I see that the American Medical Association is a powerful lobbying force and many policy makers may like the idea of having their own doctors. The fight over this issue will be hard fought and long. As it stands at this writing, this is becoming a rapidly growing option for those patients who can afford these services.

4. Shared Medical Appointments – Shared medical appointments are
   at the other end of the continuum of concierge medicine. Shared
   medical appointments are now being conducted at many large
   medical centers. These appointments involve several patients
   meeting at the same time. The number of patients can vary, but
   can range from 6 to 20 patients at one time. There may be one to
   three doctors, a nurse and a social worker who will see and talk to
   the patients during their appointments. The doctor will interview
   a patient in front of the other patients and will provide disease
   and health maintenance information to the patient being inter-
   viewed as well as the other patients in the room. The patients are
   asked to share any questions, problems or experiences in front of
   other patients in order to provide an environment of sharing and
   learning among all patients involved. Physical exams, if needed,
   are conducted behind a curtain in the same room. Shared medical
   appointments generally last about 90 minutes with patients being
   allowed to leave earlier if they need to and/or don't want to stay and
   learn from other patients.

The theory behind the shared medical appointments is that it
allows the physician to see three times or more the number of
patients he would be able to see one on one. The other theories are
that shared medical appointments cut costs and provide patients
with access to more medical personnel in a shorter period of time.
The nurse and social worker can address issues that need to be
addressed at the same time that the doctor is interviewing other
patients. The goal, of course, is to provide greater access to the
services and a higher level of patient education and support.

The advantages to shared medical appointments can be numerous
according to early feedback. Once patients get over the shock of
sharing personal information with a roomful of strangers, they
report a higher level of understanding about their disease processes
and medical management. They also have stated that they felt
less alone in their medical situations after hearing other patients'
struggles and accomplishments. The other advantage stated was
that they were able to get into see the physician more quickly. The

patients also reported that they felt they were with the physician as long or longer than they would have been with an individual appointment.

The major disadvantage with shared medical appointments is, of course, a loss of privacy. The other concern expressed by some patients is that there is a loss of individuality in the treatment options and concern that the physician is not focusing on them when preparing a treatment plan. For those patients concerned about privacy issues and protecting their medical history, shared medical appointments are probably not going to be the best option. Patients who are not that concerned about protecting their medical histories may find shared medical appointments a more efficient way of getting into see physicians, especially those physicians who are in specialty areas with limited availability.

5. Corporate takeovers of physician practices- A trend that is already being seen is the takeover of individual physician practices by hospitals and health care corporations. The advantages to this trend are that the physicians can take advantage of billing services, marketing, patient referrals and office staffing. The disadvantages are that the corporations and hospitals can tack on additional fees, can set the number of patients the physicians see during the course of a day and place limitations on their practices and policies. This is a trend that I have personally seen very little patient benefit from. Costs are generally higher, patient time with doctors is usually decreased and physicians start resenting their lack of control over their practices.

6. Increased reliance on Health Advocates – As health care resources dwindle and competition for adequate health care increases, patients are going to be looking for additional ways to navigate health care and get the most out of their health care encounters. A Health Advocate can increase your safety in the health care system; can reduce your overall health care costs and provide a reliable resource for information and health care planning. The disadvantage of using a Health Advocate is the initial added expense.

Advocates do charge fees for their services, but you can often compensate for this additional cost through long term health care service savings.

The trends mentioned above are, no doubt, just the tip of the iceberg in the ever changing health care landscape. As a patient, it will be vitally important to keep up with the trends and options that are available. Unlike in the long ago past when health care was affordable and accessible to most, the future is going to see many rapid changes. As a health care consumer, it will be necessary to carefully study the proposals being discussed in the political realms. Get your information from non-biased, thorough sources. Write your government representatives and vote to make sure that your voice is heard in the reshaping of American health care.

As a patient, be involved in your care. Don't be afraid to ask questions and to question your health care providers. Be responsible in your health care decisions. It is your life, your body and your quality of life at stake. No one will care more about your health than you do. Most importantly, make lifestyle changes necessary to enhance your overall health, follow proper preventative health care recommendations and screenings and live healthily and happily.

Index

A

E

G

H

N

O

S